A guide to starting your own Complementary Therapy practice

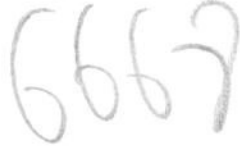

Vision without action is a daydream
Action without vision is a nightmare

Japanese proverb

For Elsevier:

Senior Commissioning Editor: Sarena Wolfaard
Associate Editor: Claire Wilson
Project Manager: Morven Dean
Design: Bruce Hogarth

A guide to starting your own Complementary Therapy practice

Elaine M Aldred
BSc (Hons) DCLicAc DipHerbMed DipCHM

Nottingham Chiropractic Clinic, Nottingham, UK

Forewords by

Martin Young BSc (Hons) BSc DC FCC MEWI
Yeovil Chiropractic Clinic, Yeovil, UK

Richard Blackwell
Principal, Northern College of Acupuncture, York, UK

CHURCHILL LIVINGSTONE

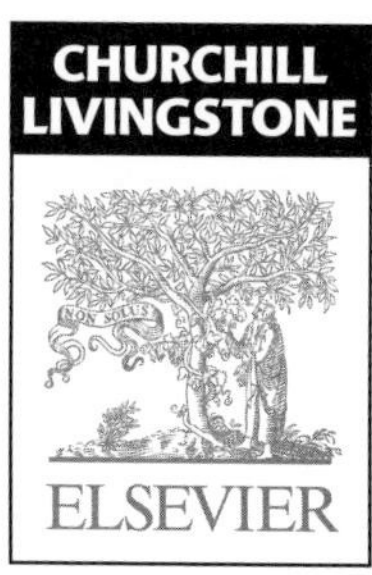

EDINBURGH LONDON NEW YORK OXFORD PHILADELPHIA ST LOUIS SYDNEY TORONTO 2007

CHURCHILL
LIVINGSTONE
An imprint of Elsevier Limited

First published 2007

ISBN-13 9780443103094

ISBN-10 0443 103097

British Library Cataloguing in Publication Data
A catalogue record for this book is available from the British Library

Library of Congress Cataloging in Publication Data
A catalog record for this book is available from the Library of Congress

Notice
Neither the Publisher nor the Author assume any responsibility for any loss or injury and/or damage to persons or property arising out of or related to any use of the material contained in this book. It is the responsibility of the treating practitioner, relying on independent expertise and knowledge of the patient, to determine the best treatment and method of application for the patient.

The Publisher

Printed in China

Contents

Part III Financial matters

Part IV Procedure

Forewords

When the author first told me she planned to prepare a book covering the essentials of business set-up for the complementary and alternative medicine (CAM) practitioner, I was delighted. Having been involved in preparing cash flow projections and researching business and marketing plans for such clinics in a previous incarnation myself, I was more than aware that the skills needed to treat patients successfully bear little or no relationship to those required to start and then manage a business. Indeed, whereas I cannot easily recall a practice that went belly-up because of a lack of clinical expertise or patient satisfaction, I know of sadly too many that failed because they were set up the wrong way, in the wrong place, with the wrong expectations, the wrong staff, the wrong financing or, most usually, the wrong combination of some or all of the above.

When, in a typically brisk and organized fashion, Elaine Aldred produced a detailed outline of what she was planning, I was immediately impressed by how good a job she was going to make of it. I can think of no other colleague who has the depth and breadth of experience required to put such a book together; not only does she have top-flight qualifications as a biochemist, chiropractor, acupuncturist, and herbalist (both western and Chinese) but she has also practised in most, if not all, of the clinical models which are discussed in the following pages. As such, she brings almost two decades of practical common sense to her writing – something that is all too often missing from generic books on such topics.

This is a book to be introduced at the undergraduate level: I can but emphasize the amount of heartache, stress and depression that could be saved if every CAM student read this book in their final year of study; however, even if you are a weathered veteran of practice, I am prepared to wager that you will learn something from listening to what Elaine is saying. That something may even be the realization that the way in which you structure, manage and run your clinic is completely wrong and has been causing you unnecessary, premature grey hairs and gastric ulcers.

There is no doubt that most practices I have come across could do with an objective review and overhaul, and the results of such action invariably improve both profitability and patient care. What you are about to read should act both as a catalyst for such change and offer friendly, practical advice as to why and how it can be achieved. It is not often that a book lives up to the soubriquet 'essential', but I can think of no CAM practitioner or student, be they working for themselves, as an associate or in full employment; seeing patients in their spare bedroom or running large, multidisciplinary group practices who should not invest in this book and absorb its detail. For some, it will be a case of 'better late than never', for some 'a stitch in time saving nine', if you are lucky you will be in the 'forewarned is forearmed' category, but by whatever route you have reached this book, the chapters that follow can only improve things for you, your practice and your patients.

Martin Young,
January 2006

It is clear that patients derive great benefit from complementary and alternative medicine. To take acupuncture as an example, both patients and practitioners report remarkable responses to treatment for a huge variety of people with a wide range of conditions. Robust research evidence is still patchy, but results are accumulating from rigorous studies demonstrating clear benefits for conditions as diverse as migraine, osteoarthritis, and menorrhagia. A consensus statement from the National Institutes of Health in the US identified good evidence of efficacy for nausea and some kinds of pain, and suggestive evidence of value in stroke rehabilitation, asthma, period pain and a wide range of musculoskeletal conditions. Practitioners would add many more to this list. It is striking, for example, that there are little reliable research data on digestive system disorders, nor on anxiety or depression, which are frequently successfully treated in practice.

A 1999 survey by the Maryland Acupuncture Society (Cassidy & Emad 2002) found that the most common reason for patients to consult an acupuncturist was a specific illness, but nearly as important was that they were 'seeking care of their whole being', and 21% were basically healthy but seeking care to stay well. Interestingly, 39% regarded their acupuncturist as their primary care provider. Repeated surveys in the US and UK also show high levels of patient satisfaction with their acupuncture treatment and the care they receive from their practitioner.

Claire Cassidy's research in the US (Cassidy & Emad 2002) casts further light on the reasons for the popularity of acupuncture, many of which probably apply to other CAM therapies as well. Of course, patients spoke about the relief of both physical and emotional/spiritual symptoms, but they also described with a high frequency a general sense of feeling better, stronger, more in control, more whole and centred. Cassidy's research also identifies very clearly the importance to patients of the tranquil atmosphere of the clinic, the rapport they have with their practitioner, and their sense of working in partnership with their practitioner. Perhaps most importantly, patients reported increases in self-awareness and body-awareness, and feeling empowered to make changes to lifestyle and self-care. Many seem to experience increased 'self-efficacy', which many studies show to be 'the single strongest factor predicting health and healing'.

Similarly, Sylvia Schroer's research in the UK (Schroer 2005) shows that patients here also describe feeling very different during and after acupuncture treatment, and being changed by it. Patients commonly experience 'an increase or decrease in energy levels and a sense of relaxation or even euphoria' during treatment. After treatment they report feeling clearer, re-balanced, cleansed. They use descriptions such as 'I know something in me has been sparked off, the body heals itself'. They also echo the US research in emphasizing the importance of their relationship with their acupuncturist, which many describe as more of a peer-to-peer relationship than they have with their medical practitioner, and they talk about the process of treatment helping them to make important life changes.

It is clear then that acupuncture, like other CAM therapies, has a great deal to offer, and that this extends well beyond the relief of symptoms. As the evidence mounts in the West, we are also seeing dramatic improvements in the standards of training of practitioners. This is particularly promoted by robust systems of professional accreditation. In the UK the work of the British Acupuncture Accreditation Board is widely regarded as an example of good practice, with its emphasis on institutional self-reflection and its developmental approach. Academic standards are also increasingly being underpinned by the validation of awards by universities. This process is not unproblematic of course, and many practitioner-educators are acutely aware of the need to maintain a broad focus on the development of the practitioner, as well as the transfer of knowledge and technical skills. Overall we are seeing better-educated practitioners going out with a wide range of personal qualities and professional skills which equip them to meet the needs of patients in profound and holistic ways.

Despite their training and all they have to give to patients, practitioners face major challenges in establishing successful practices. Most are self-employed and many are naturally more interested in their healing work than in the business aspects of their practice. Yet sound financial planning, good marketing and robust business systems are critical. Without them, the most talented practitioners can fail to reach out to the patients they could be helping, and this is a tragic waste for all concerned. Although business skills are increasingly covered in practitioner education, they inevitably still comprise a small part of the overall curriculum, and often the need for them is not fully appreciated until the new practitioners are establishing their first practice. The transition into practice over the first few years can be very challenging and it takes time to build up the word of mouth networks of personal recommendation which underpin a mature and successful practice. Even when this stage is reached, a sound business base is essential. Practitioners need to do more than make a living from their practice, they need to continue to learn and develop. This may be by undertaking self study or new courses and seminars, by regular supervision, or by structured processes of rigorous reflection on practice. Ideally it will involve a combination of all these, and these activities can only be supported by a successful practice and a good income. Then the practitioners will thrive, and their healing work with their patients will benefit. So there is a great need for Elaine Aldred's comprehensive and supportive book on the business aspects of CAM practice. I welcome it and I hope it will contribute to the flowering of many successful practices, taking to the public all the benefits which CAM therapies have to offer.

Richard Blackwell

Cassidy C, Emad M 2002 What patients say about Chinese medicine. In: Cassidy C (ed) Contemporary Chinese medicine and acupuncture. Churchill Livingstone, New York

Schroer S 2005 Patients' explanatory models of acupuncture: how and why do they think it works? European Journal of Oriental Medicine 5(1):34–43

Preface

This book has been written from my own trial-and-error experiences and extensive conversations with colleagues, students and newly qualified practitioners. The general view is that the complementary profession has still not fully got to grips with the subject of business skills. When I left Chiropractic College there were no business studies built into the curriculum, and this left me floundering in confusion as to how to begin my own venture. Business skills are, thankfully, something that many complementary educational establishments or professional bodies are now trying to address.

I have worked in several, varied, settings: from home, from a spacious clinic replete with staff and X-ray equipment, from a licensed room at a GP's surgery, from a podiatrist's clinic and from a squash club. It has certainly been a voyage of discovery to find the setting that is entirely suited to my lifestyle and needs.

It is unlikely that any profession in the world is able to compete with the field of complementary medicine for the diversity of its practitioners; some entering straight from school, others choosing it as a second career later on in life, with a wealth of life experience behind them. Despite their differences, they are all linked by their desire to help people and their unlimited enthusiasm.

Almost all practitioners will at some point want to work for themselves, whether immediately after qualifying or in the fullness of time when they have gained enough experience to be confident in branching out on their own.

The complementary field allows for the provision of the same level of excellence in the smallest unit of one person established in a modest set-up as in a large multipractitioner clinic.

The choice of set-up can leave practitioners quite bewildered, rendering them almost catatonic with indecision while they try to rationalize all the options and deal with the complexities of the marketing and financial skills required for even the most modest of situations. Trying to avoid falling foul of the various pieces of legislation and legal requirements (which change on a regular basis) can seem an impossible task.

If you have not thought the process through in detail before establishing your practice, you may then find yourself in a situation not ideally suited to your needs. Making changes at that stage can be very difficult. Having said this, be prepared to accept that it is not unusual for you to have to revise your situation when circumstances change, with the arrival of children, for example. Behind every successful clinic is a therapist who has had the flexibility of attitude to adapt as circumstances demanded.

Direction is all-important. To wander aimlessly through the process of setting up your own clinic without any goals or timetable is a recipe for disaster, financial and emotional. You have to plan its conception as precisely as you would a treatment.

A great deal of dedication is required, regardless of your choice of lifestyle. Complementary medicine is not likely to make you a multimillionaire, but handled properly will give you a good income and an entirely satisfying way of life.

You are working within an area that you have chosen and has not been thrust upon you. It is therefore something that you enjoy doing, that will allow you to practise all the knowledge you have acquired during your education and will hopefully encourage you to learn more.

This book is designed to overcome the confusion of opening a new clinic, for both new and established practitioners. It will guide you in a logical manner through the process so that you can achieve your dream of self-sufficiency in your chosen therapy. If you feel confident in certain subjects then it is possible to skip to the areas that you find most helpful. In certain areas where information is constantly changing (e.g. legislation and tax rules) you are given advice on where to look for up-to-the-minute answers.

Although many complementary professions state that their customers are clients not patients, I will continue to call them patients. As regulation, certainly in the UK, is on its way and the various professions are serious in their intent to treat, I feel that it is more appropriate to use the term patient.

In order to avoid gender bias, when it has been necessary to write about a single patient, practitioner or other professional, the person is referred to as as 'he' in some chapters and 'she' in others on a strictly alternating basis.

As I am a UK practitioner and have practised all my professional working life within the UK, I naturally have a grasp of the legal and financial environment of my native country and the majority of the text is thus written from a UK perspective. However, do not let this put you off if you are practising in another country. The processes practitioners go through to set up their own practice are remarkably similar regardless of what part of the world they intend to practice in. This was brought home to me while researching the various elements of business start-up in Australia, Canada, New Zealand and the USA. Many of the aspects of marketing and producing a business plan described in this book have come from reading countless examples from other countries and adapting them to the needs of the complementary healthcare profession. I have included, at the end of chapters, relevant websites for the above countries in addition to those for the UK.

Wherever you decide to establish your practice, with the population displaying an ever-increasing enthusiasm for complementary medicine there has never been a better time to start your own clinic.

Elaine M Aldred
March 2006

Acknowledgements

I would like to acknowledge my gratitude to the Northern College of Acupuncture and the Anglo European College of Chiropractic for allowing me access to their students while writing this book. The input from the students greatly assisted in fine-tuning certain elements of the book.

Richard Blackwell and Martin Young for providing me with opportunities which have made it possible for me to develop in an entirely unexpected direction.

I would also like to thank the staff of the Holywell Annexe Clinic and my colleague Anne Etherton for patiently dealing with various phone calls to clarify minutiae, so necessary when compiling data.

Mr William Barnes for the useful and rapidly returned emails.

My father Edwin who made life so much easier in preparing the financial calculations, and make it possible for me to have the space to write this book.

My son Alexander for giving the incentive to make me see that it was possible to change the course of my life.

Most of all I appreciate the emotional and logistic support given to me by my mother Sheila, without whom I definitely would not be where I am today.

Part 1

Initial preparation

Where do I start? Brainstorming

1

Chapter contents

You have just qualified or have completed a clinical placement, and have a burning desire to strike out on your own. You have an appreciation that having your own clinic amounts to more than just treating patients, but how do you begin to make your dream reality?

The biggest decision

First of all you have to decide whether striking out on your own is for you.

Before you even start working your way through the mechanics of what premises, equipment and finance you will need, you must be clear about whether this course of action is right for you and what you want out of it. To do this you must ask yourself some very important questions and answer them honestly.

Life mapping

Many people wander through life with no clear idea of what they want to do and as a consequence where they are going. In other words, they lack direction. They do not enjoy their work and experience a constant need for escape. Of those who do try to set up their own business, some may then live in a permanent state of crisis management and confusion, and as a result are still unfulfilled. This situation is even less desirable when it finally spills over into their private life.

You do not want to live this way and have already made a very large step in the right direction by choosing to study to become a practitioner of complementary medicine. So, to continue in your positive start, you need to have an overall view of where you are going now you have qualified. To help you obtain this, ask yourself the following questions:

- Where do you want to be in 5, 10, 20 years' time?
- What kind of lifestyle do you want?

These questions should lay the groundwork for your strategic thinking, an overview of your life. The answers you come up with should be viewed as a guide but are in no way inflexible. Situations will change over the years when other factors will enter your life, for example you may have children if you do not already have them. Such factors may alter or vary the main thread, but you will be able to actively decide how to make this alteration productive, because you have a reference point to work from.

Your character

The next ingredient you need to assess is yourself.

You must be able to see yourself as others see you. This is important for two reasons:

1. Your everyday life involves close interactions with people in a one-to-one working relationship, either with a patient, colleague or member of staff.
2. You must work in a situation that is best suited to you.

It is an unfortunate fact that many people are blissfully unaware of how they appear to the world at large, of their shortcomings and, most importantly of all, their good points.

You need to know truthfully what sort of person you are so that you end up in the best possible working environment for you and, if necessary, address any personal character flaws and build on your positive points along the way.

Personality

As self-reflection is an important part of being a practitioner, the following exercises may help to give you the right perspective on the type of person you really are, and how suitable you will be for your intended course of action and starting to organize your life map.

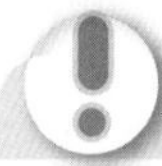

Exercise 1

Write out on paper how you see yourself and ask someone whose opinion you value and who you can rely upon to be honest, how she feels the world at large perceives you.

Be as honest about yourself as you can be. The way in which you feel comfortable working depends on your personality.

Exercise 2

Next you need to be able to gauge your suitability for the project ahead. Again, brainstorm with someone you trust and who is prepared to give you an unbiased opinion. You need a balanced viewpoint, since you will be committing a great deal of time, effort and, over a period of years, money to your practice.

These are some general questions you can ask:

What motivates you? Are you self-motivated or does motivation have to come from someone else? You will have to be highly motivated to run your own clinic.

Do you respond better when you become caught up in situations? You may not be able to cope with the steady pace of working from home.

Are you hard working and goal-directed? You have to clarify this regardless of the size of clinic, since this quality is necessary for good clinical practice. In a large clinic, however, where overheads are high, this aspect can be added to your managerial skills.

Are you persistent and dynamic? You will have to be if you want to run a big clinic.

What financial risks are you prepared to take? If the answer is very few then you are more suited to a small set-up, probably mobile, working from home or from a licensed room.

What is your comfort zone in the amount of stress you can take? If you do not respond well to stress then do not be overambitious in your plans.

Are you well organized and able to plan? You may well be able to handle a large clinic if the answer is yes.

Are you a problem solver? This is a skill you will naturally require as a practitioner, but a larger set-up requires this on a day-to-day basis. The larger a clinic you have, the more variables are involved.

Do you have any management skills? If you decide to have staff or other practitioners working in your clinic, you will need to be able to relate well to them and quickly resolve any problems that arise.

Are you a leader and motivator of others? Running a large enterprise requires someone who is able to take charge and inspire others to perform well.

How well do you work with others? If you run a large clinic you must enjoy having other practitioners around you. The same goes for your having a room in a multidisciplinary clinic, where you will probably have to do a room share with another practitioner. If you do not like having people in your working space, then consider working as a sole practitioner from your own premises.

Do you like working flat out or do you want a more relaxed approach to give you more time to think? If you intend to finish up with a large clinic, then the overheads will ensure that you have to work at a fast pace, unless you are in the unusual position of having other practitioners working for you covering these costs and more.

Are you excited by the cut and thrust of running a business and can you cope with the pressure? Someone who likes this type of situation is well suited to running a large establishment. If you cannot cope with pressure then consider a small, manageable practice.

Do you want to spend as little time as possible travelling or do you prefer to have some distance between the cocoon of home and the bustle of the workplace? Do not forget that as a therapist you only earn money when you work, and travel time cuts down the number of patients you may be able to see in a day. Travel may also take up time you need with your family.

Do you have any skills you can take from your last occupation? For example, midwives may be in an excellent position to specialize in mother and baby treatment, giving them a clear idea of the area in which they may eventually wish to specialize.

How are you going to view the time generated by the gaps between treatments when you first start out? This is a wonderful opportunity for planning and learning and may be the only time you get to do this in your career. If you are going to worry endlessly about where the next patient is coming from it may be a good idea to start from a low-cost practice at home or in a licensed room.

How are you going to cope if you are not financially able to give up your current job to pursue your new career? It is very likely that you will have to build up a practice in unsocial hours while holding down your full-time job, unless you have considerable interest-free backing behind you. It is not easy to come home from one job to start on another, and makes for a long day. Your weekends may also have to be sacrificed, depending on how fast you want to build your practice.

Could you give up your full-time job and look for one that is less challenging and less well paid but covers the cost of living while you build up your practice? If you are able to do this and live within a tight budget, going without certain luxuries you are used to, then you may have more psychological contentment and a sensible compromise.

Exercise 3

Write a list in two columns. Make a note of the aspects that you would like to experience in your life and business and another stating what you would dislike and not want to experience as part of your life. This will give you something to refer back to when you start to look at the type of practice you want to run.

Blend these questions and viewpoints with trying to define your motivation for wanting your own clinic. If it is just because you are fed up working for someone then you may have to analyse why this is. A well-defined start makes for clarity of vision.

Here are a few reasons practitioners gave for wanting to start their own practice and which you may want to consider for your own situation.

Autonomy. You become the decision maker in treating cases and are master of your own destiny.

Flexibility and independence. When you are your own boss you can choose where you work, when you work and how you work. For instance, if as a practitioner you have children then the working hours can fit around them. Do not forget, however, that the larger a clinic becomes the less flexible the working hours may be.

Earning capacity. There is a mistaken belief that running your own clinic immediately increases your income, since the money goes straight into your pocket and not into that of someone else. Do not forget that, if you work for someone else, your employer will be covering the running costs of the business. You will now have to do this.

Challenge. The practitioner wants an occupation with constant challenges and a permanent environment of growth and self-improvement.

Pride. You can take pride in you achievements with patients.

Status. Some practitioners enjoy the status of being in charge.

Leadership. This may well relate to status and pride, since practitioners envision themselves at the head of a clinic where they are overseeing an integrated group of practitioners, achieving remarkable results.

Joining a professional body

This is something you may have automatically done, since most courses are in some way affiliated with professional bodies.

It is a false economy to feel that it is not worthwhile, since there are usually reasonably priced new-member packages and in may cases allowances for struggling practitioners on a low income. The more prestigious and well known the association, the more beneficial you will find the cost of your membership. They are there to support you, to link you to your therapeutic community, so that you do not feel isolated.

If you are not sure, then all the leading associations have a website from which you can get preliminary information, and their membership secretaries are usually very helpful in answering queries. You need to know what type of services they have on offer. Services such as counselling, legal advice, legal support, and advice on ethics may be available.

A professional body should be easily approachable and available to their members. If they do not have permanent staff, how fast do they reply to your call? Can they easily answer all your questions?

Find out the numbers of members in the associations. The associations with more people will have more of a voice and also more cash to use for the benefit and support of their members.

Professional associations are also a vital link with what is happening to the status of the respective disciplines, by representing their members over contentious issues and keeping information flowing; for example, if new legislation is being put into place, or if any product their members are currently using becomes banned.

Look at the advertising they have been performing for the whole profession. Does it look professional?

Professional advisors

There is a large amount of helpful information on the Internet. Professional advisors for new business can be found at places such as enterprise agencies, local government, business links, chambers of commerce, The Prince's Trust.

In some cases, initial consultations may be free of charge.

Having made your decision

You are establishing your own clinic because you want to be your own boss. No matter what the size of the establishment you eventually wish to be the proprietor of, the fundamental principles of running a practice apply to all situations.

All decisions, right or wrong, are made by you, and problems associated with the practice are nobody's problems but yours. To a certain extent, even if you work for someone else, you have been making clinical decisions on your own. Going entirely on your own is merely the next step.

If you are someone who enjoys treating patients and cannot bear the thought of having to deal with administrative matters outside clinical practice then going it alone is not for you.

Be prepared to accept that you may make mistakes during your business life. Behind every successful clinic is a therapist who has learned by the mistakes she has made and who has not given up at the first hurdle.

This is also the time when you must work out strategies and organize yourself so that you will not be caught out be any administrative or financial surprises when you become busy.

Most importantly, do not forget that you have a life outside of work.

Useful websites

Australia

http://www.acci.asn.au/

Australian Chamber of Commerce and Industry

http://www.aiia.com.au/i-cms.isp?page=850

Australian Industry Information Association

http://www.business.gov.au/Business+Entry+Point/

Australian Government
Business.gov.au offers the initial information you will need to start your own business.

http://www.youngaustralians.org/

Foundation for Young Australians

Canada

Many websites are bilingual.

http://bsa.cbsc.org/gol/bsa/site.nsf/en/index.html

Canadian government's start-up assistant
This covers all the territories.

http://canada.gc.ca/main_e.html

Canadian Government

http://www.cra-arc.gc.ca/

Canadian Revenue Agency
Very helpful website to guide you through the tax system of different methods of trading, as well as many tax issues. All the guides and forms you will ever need are also available on the website for you to save and print out.

http://www.cybf.ca/

Canadian Youth Business Foundation

The Canadian Youth Business Foundation is a national charitable organization that assists young Canadian entrepreneurs, age 18–34, to start up their own business.

New Zealand

Governmental websites are bilingual.

http://www.biz.org.nz/public/home.aspx?sectionid=53

Business Information Zone (BIZ)
Small Business information website by the New Zealand Government. Very comprehensive site covering a wide range of topics on starting your own business, even running a business from home.

http://www.govt.nz/

New Zealand Government

UK

http://www.adviceguide.org.uk/

Citizens' Advice Bureau

http://www.businesslink.gov.uk/

Business Link

http://www.chamberonline.co.uk/

British Chamber of Commerce

http://www.dti.gov.uk/

Department of Trade and Industry

http://www.nfea.com/

National Federation of Enterprise Agencies

http://www.princes-trust.org.uk/

The Prince's Trust

http://www.sbs.gov.uk/

Small Business Service

http://www.sfedi.co.uk/

Small Firms Enterprise Development Initiative

http://www.smallbusinessadvice.org.uk/

Small Business Advice

USA

http://www.business.gov/

Business.gov
This is probably more user friendly for the uninitiated.

http://www.dol.gov/osbp/

Department of Labor, Office of Small Business Programs

http://www.firstgov.gov/

United States Government
Website with useful information, with linkages to all the states.

http://www.irs.gov/businesses/small/content/0,,id=98864,00.html

Internal Revenue Service
Website providing a page of useful links to the various state websites with relevant information for businesses.

http://www.sba.gov/

United States Small Business Administration
This site links up to the various states and offices that assist small businesses locally.

How do you decide on the type of practice you want?

2

Chapter contents

Having gone through the stage of assessing your personality and goals in life, it is now time to review the different ways of practising.

Mobile practice

This is probably the simplest way to set up.

Advantages

- *Low running costs.*
- *Keeps work nicely separated from home.*
- *Patients who are unable to leave their homes can be treated.*
- *Cost of travel, wear and tear on the car, etc., can be built into the cost of the treatment.*

Disadvantages

- *Transport.* You will need a car to transport you and your equipment. The insurance on your car will have to be changed, as the vehicle will be classed as being used for business.

- *Injury.* If any of the equipment is heavy, such as a treatment couch, then you might injure yourself. This will mean that you will be limited in the equipment you can use, as it should not be too heavy to lift.
- *Personal security.* You will be going to somewhere you do not know on the first visit and are relying on your patient being legitimate.
- *Inefficient use of time.* You will need to allow more time between appointments than you would if you were seeing patients in static premises.
- *Poor financial return.* Usually home visits take time, since you will need to get there and unload and load the car, which will limit the number of patients you can see in a day. House calls are largely made to people who are housebound through some form of disability. This might mean that they have a lower income than the rest of the population and are without much available spare cash for your treatment, so the amount they will be able to pay will be limited.
- *Less control over working environment.*
- *This type of practice will take a long time to build up.*

Locum work

Advantages

- *Instant patients.*
- *No financial responsibility.*

Disadvantages

- *Difficult to take over someone else's patient load,* particularly if the patients are aware that it is a temporary situation.
- *May never get to see completion of a treatment.*
- *Contractual clause preventing work within a certain radius.*
- *Work may be spasmodic.* This will make it difficult to obtain a smooth flow of income, leading to less financial security.

Working with a particular sports team

Advantages

- *Low financial commitment.* Equipment may be supplied. Will not need premises.
- *Opportunity for immersion in an interest.* Get to travel with the team, and see the sport first hand.
- *Gain invaluable experience with sports injuries.* If this is your interest then it will open opportunities to become a specialist in the field.

Disadvantages

- *Difficult field to break into.*
- *Commitment of time is very high.* As the teams travel a great deal you will also have to do so. You may be required to go with them at a moment's notice.
- *You may be tied to one team.* Generally teams like to have your services exclusively.
- *Financial gain may not be high.* Only large teams can afford to pay generously for a therapist. Those therapists who are deemed to be very important in dealing quickly with injuries will take priority.

Spas

Advantages

- *Low cost.* Equipment is generally supplied.
- *Professional set-up.* These places are usually decorated and furnished well and carefully maintained.
- *Patients are committed to their health.*

Disadvantages

- *You may not be able to work at a pace suitable for you.* Even if you are self-employed you may have to pay the spa a fairly large fee to be there or they may be taking a percentage of your earnings off you. You may well end up in a situation where you are required to operate a high-volume practice, working at a much higher rate than you feel comfortable with. You are also there for the convenience of the spa's customers and appointments may be sporadic.
- *You may not be allowed to be self-employed.* This will negate your independence, the reason why you trained in the first place. As well as having your hours dictated to you, there may also be an exclusion clause in the contract preventing you from working elsewhere within a certain radius.
- *You may be required to sell products.* The spa functions to make a profit, and products are the way they make money.

Working from home

This is another cost-effective ways of setting up a practice. It is the way many practitioners start and continue their working life.

Advantages

- *Relaxed atmosphere.* You are in your own home.
- *Complete control of work environment.*

- *On-site staff and chaperone.* Your family may be available to assist you in a few of the administrative requirements of a clinic. Another person in the vicinity makes for a reduction in indecent assault accusations and increases personal safety.
- *Flexible working hours.* Practitioners may be more comfortable working outside the nine-to-five scenario. Certain family requirements such as school pick-ups can be easily catered for. It will also enable you to see more of your family. The market may demand a period of treating outside normal working hours. You will be able to accommodate this, as you can dictate the hours you work.
- *Working at your own pace.* Immediately you rent or buy premises your workload has to go up to cover the increased expenses.
- *No need to travel.* Work is on site so there will be no fighting with the rush hour traffic. If you are in a position where transport is difficult, then working from home solves this problem.
- *Tax.* There will be many items in your home you may be able to offset against tax, e.g. part of gas and electricity bills.

Disadvantages

- *Distractions.* These are more likely at home and may involve unexpected visitors in the treatment room such as small children and pets. The noise generated by a household will affect the ambience of professionalism.
- *May affect the freedom of your family.* Your family will not be able to relax in their own home since they will have to stay away from the treatment room and remain quiet while patients are in.
- *Encroachment of clinic into the home environment.* The clinic phone will have to be kept separate from the personal phone. Any calls made from the home phone should be dialled using the code to withhold your number. It has not been unknown for a patient to ring 1471 to find out where the practitioner has called from.
- *Patients may appear at the house at any time requesting treatment.* You have to be firm with patients about hours of work, or they may try to take advantage of you.
- *Restrictions.* Neighbours may object to the amount of people coming and going from your house. There may be a covenant on the house preventing you from running a business. Planning permission should be sought before attempting to open up in your home. It is unlikely that it will be refused if you keep to the guidelines that allow you to use a room in your home for business purposes. It is always more difficult to consult with the Local Authority planning office for retrospective permission after a problem has been encountered.
- *Appearance may not be professional.* Your home will have to be very tidy, with the areas where patients are likely to go in good repair and decoration. Some patients will always prefer being treated in a clinical environment.

- *May be difficult to maintain confidentiality.* If you have to have patients waiting outside the room, they may be able to hear through the door. The same problem will go for anyone in your house.
- *Potential accusations of indecent assault.* Some practitioners ensure that there is always someone in the house when they are treating a patient and that the patient is made aware of this.
- *Increased risk of theft.* Increased security may be required both internally and externally. Burglar alarms may have to be fitted, since you will be announcing when you are away because you need to let your patients know about it.
- *Can be isolating.* It can be very lonely if you live alone. As a sole practitioner there will only be opportunities for interactions with other practitioners at conferences and meetings.
- *Extra insurance.* The home policy will have to be altered to cover public liability, and equipment.

Renting

Rooms

This is a very common way of starting out, usually done under licence.

Advantages

- *Low cost.* You may only be required to pay for the time you are there, or pay a percentage of your earnings. There should be no added costs for payments for rates, electricity, etc.
- *No responsibilities.* Whoever you rent the room from will have to maintain the premises and perform any repairs.
- *Good supply of potential patients.* If there is more than one type of practitioner, then patients in the waiting room may also need your services.
- *Professional networking.* In a multidisciplinary practice there is an opportunity to forge professional links.
- *Useful association with reputable practitioners.*
- *Receptionist or someone to answer calls.* If part of the receptionist's job is also to handle the money, then this saves time and allows you to see more patients.
- *Simple contract.* This is usually in the form of a licence, which is a simple contract. There is typically a short lead-time, often a month, during which each party can give notice. The contract can be easily renegotiated.
- *Possibility of working from more than one clinic.* This will enable you to build up a larger range of patients. You need to check that the contract you have with each clinic allows you to do this.

Disadvantages

- *No security.* You might lose your situation at a moment's notice.
- *No control over rent increases.*
- *No say in the room decoration or appearance.*
- *You will not be able to make the room your own if you are sharing it.*
- *Personal conflicts with other practitioners and staff.*
- *May not get a fair share of patients.* Sometimes receptionists can be biased, ensuring that patients are offered to certain practitioners first.
- *If you are not working with practitioners who have a good reputation, it may be assumed that you are also of the same standard.*

Premises

Advantages

- *More security.* Contracts tend to be for a few years, allowing you greater stability when building your clinic. There is more control over rent increases, which can be negotiated before signing the contract.
- *You have more say in how the place is run.* It will be your clinic, therefore you get to make all the decisions on how it is run.
- *Control over decoration and appearance.*
- *Other people working for you.* You may be able to bring in extra income by having other practitioners in your clinic.

Disadvantages

- *May require permission for change of use.* If the premises are not currently in use as a clinic, then planning permission for change of usage will be required.
- *Requires long-term commitment.* This may create problems if the business is not going well and you need to get yourself a less expensive set-up. You will still be expected to continue to pay the rent until you find someone to take it over.
- *Required to perform repairs and maintenance.* You may be required to perform general repairs yourself, such as dealing with plumbing problems, etc. There is a type of lease called a fully repairing lease, in which case you will have to perform repairs to the fabric of the building or the ground it is occupying.
- *Will have to cover the cost of utilities.* It is unlikely that electricity, gas, etc. will be covered in the rental.
- *Reduces saleability.* When you want to retire or sell the clinic, you will only be able to sell the equipment and the goodwill. This may make it harder to sell. All the money you paid in rent is effectively dead money, since you have nothing to show for it.

Buying your own place

Advantages

- *Clinic and premises entirely under your control.* You have total autonomy. No one but you has a say in how things are run. Choice of furnishings and décor is entirely under your control. Apart from planning permission and building regulations, there are no restrictions on any changes you may wish to make to the building.
- *Complete security.* Providing you are able to pay for the premises or are able to keep up any mortgage repayments, you can occupy them for as long as you wish.
- *Asset for sale.* The ownership of the premises will be a large bargaining chip when it comes to the sale of the clinic. If there are possibilities for living on site, this will also increase saleability.
- *Possibilities of extra income.* The other rooms or a section of the building can be rented out.

Disadvantages

- *Expensive start-up and running costs.* Unless you have substantial capital behind you, you will be committed to a hefty mortgage repayment. This will account for a large part of your outgoings. Equipment, furnishing and decoration will add to the cost. All the utilities will have to be paid for.
- *May have to get planning permission for change of usage.* The property may have been used for something else before and the new business may need permission to operate from it.
- *Health and safety legislation etc. may mean substantial changes to the building.* As the clinic is to be used by the general public, several alterations to the building may be needed to make it comply with regulations.

Buying an existing clinic

Many of the advantages and disadvantages are similar to those of buying your own premises and starting from scratch.

Advantages

- *Instant supply of patients.*
- *Credibility if the previous practitioner was good.*
- *Short-term financial gain if the business is productive.*

Disadvantages

- *Can be difficult to match the previous practitioner's level of expertise and style.* The complementary profession can be very personality driven and a new practitioner may be difficult for patients to accept. Therefore you may end up initially losing patients.

Conclusion

After reading this chapter you should compare the various scenarios with the assessment of how you see yourself and your aspirations.

You should now have a better idea of the way you will start to work.

It is possible to work in more than one scenario, for example some practitioners have a practice at home and rent a room in a multidisciplinary clinic. This gives them a certain amount of flexibility on working hours and a higher profile working at an established clinic where there is a good flow of patients and referrals.

Ways of trading

3

Chapter contents

Having decided the style of clinic you would like to establish, you will have to decide the manner in which you are going to trade. Each way of trading has different tax advantages and complexity.

Sole trader

This is the more usual way for therapists to run their practice.

Advantages

- *Complete control over how the practice is run.* You have no one to answer to but yourself.
- *Simple to set up.* Trading in this way requires very little organization. You will need to notify HM Revenue & Customs (a recent amalgamation of the Inland Revenue and HM Customs and Excise). If you are in a profession that is not exempt from VAT, then you will also have to inform them if you are likely to exceed the VAT limit for the year.
- *Very little administration.* Your accounts will be simple and will only be required for an audit if you incur an investigation by HM Revenue & Customs.
- *You take all the profits.*

Disadvantages

- *Personally liable for all losses.* Creditors will come after you for all your debts, and any assets such as your house, car, furniture, can be used to pay those debts.
- *May be difficult to get a loan or mortgage.* Most lenders will want to see at least 3 years of accounts to ensure that you are not a credit risk.
- *Can be very lonely.* No one is there to give you assistance in an emergency.

Limited company

You are likely to operate this way if you are taking on board a large project such as a big multidisciplinary clinic which may incur some financial risk, or you are making such a large profit that it is more financially viable to do so.

It is always advisable to employ an accountant and a solicitor to help you through this process.

Advantages

- *Financial risk is no longer personal.* The type of asset that creditors can take off you is limited to the business and what it owns. Your home and personal belongings will now be secure if your business does not go well.

Disadvantages

- *The rules regarding tax can complicated and can change from time to time.* There are also special rules for small companies.
- *You are required to file an annual return to Companies House.*

Partnership

This arrangement, when it works, can be immensely beneficial for the participants. When it goes wrong, it can be fraught with problems. Rather like a marriage, until you get into it you have no idea whether it is going to work.

It is therefore very important that you go into a partnership for all the right reasons. If you are just too lacking in motivation to work as a sole trader or are just too frightened to take your intended project on board yourself, think carefully about taking part in a partnership. Insecurity is a recipe for disaster.

If you are going into a partnership with a friend or someone close, consider carefully whether this blurring of boundaries is likely to cause a problem.

A partnership is what it suggests, everything that is done is to represent both or all of you. None of you should be looking at it as a springboard to self-promotion.

Advantages

- *Costs can be shared.* This will allow for a bigger budget than could be afforded by a sole trader.
- *One practitioner's weakness may be another's strength.* One partner may be an excellent therapist, another have outstanding business acumen. One type of therapy may handsomely compliment another, giving more effective treatment.
- *Working times can be shared.* This will allow more flexibility because the clinic can be kept open longer, therefore increasing available working hours.
- *Administration can be shared.* This is very useful if you have a large clinic, as the paperwork can be extensive.
- *Holiday cover.* There is a commitment to the clinic from each of the partners, ensuring that when one is on holiday the others will ensure everything is working smoothly and will have the authority to deal with any problems that occur.
- *More energy.* As the load and stress are shared, each partner should have more energy for work and family.
- *National Insurance is lower.*
- *No requirement to file an annual return to Companies House.*

Disadvantages

- *May be costly to set up.* It is imperative that a solicitor is hired to draw up a contract. The more complex the contract, the more expensive it will be.
- *Each partner may have different commitments and viewpoints.* One partner may end up carrying a larger load than originally intended. When anything is done, all partners have to agree to it. It they are not all of like mind, this may cause a dispute.
- *The circumstances of each partner may change.* This factor may bring about difficulties for the partnership.
- *Unless there is a written contract, each partner is responsible for the actions of the other.* If one partner is unable to pay his share, the others will have to make up the deficit. The financial difficulty of one partner may affect the others.

Setting up a partnership

A solicitor must be engaged to draft the agreement, since it must be very clear. Although this adds to the expense of the set-up, it is very important to ensure that every eventuality is covered. Disintegrations in partnership are very common. If this happens a partner may have to be bought out, or a partner may have to be prevented from selling his part of the company or contents without the others' permission.

A partnership contract should include:

- The nature of their ongoing involvement.
- What to expect if the business is sold or the partnership breaks down.

Some of the items to cover in a partnership agreement are:

- When the partnership started.
- What the business is.
- Who the partners are.
- If there is a senior partner, who it is and how that person is chosen.
- How partners can be added.
- How partners can leave.
- What happens to the departing partner's share in the business.
- What each partner has contributed in money, skill, equipment or time.
- Allocation of jobs and commitment requirements of each partner. The books, maintenance, banking have to be kept up to date. If one partner never turns up to work, then the partnership becomes uneven.
- Whether the partners may continue to work outside the partnership.
- The distribution of profits and loss within the partnership.
- What happens on death or retirement.
- How disputes are resolved.

Limited liability partnership (LLP)

This avoids the insecurity of having unlimited personal liability and being obliged to meet your partners' financial shortcomings. It has all the benefits of partnerships, including the tax advantages, but limits the liability of each individual partner.

To create one of these, you will need to complete an incorporation document, pay a fee and register the name at Companies House. An annual return will also have to be filed.

Conclusion

The way you want to work is very much linked to how you want the practice to be established.

If a partnership is involved a personality profile of each person is a must. More than one person owning a clinic immediately increases variables.

Regardless of how practitioners finally decide to trade (sole practitioner, in partnership, etc.) they will always need an accountant. Not to use an accountant is likely to be very unwise.

Useful websites

Australia

http://www.ato.gov.au/

Australian Taxation Office

http://www.business.gov.au/Business+Entry+Point/

Australian Government
For information on ways of trading.

Canada

Many websites are bilingual.

http://bsa.cbsc.org/gol/bsa/site.nsf/en/index.html

Canadian government's start-up assistant

http://www.cra-arc.gc.ca/

Canadian Revenue Agency

New Zealand

Governmental websites are bilingual.

http://www.biz.org.nz/public/content.aspx?sectionid=81&contentid=1256

Biz.org
Website on different ways of trading.

http://www.ird.govt.nz/

New Zealand Inland Revenue

UK

http://www.hmrc.gov.uk/

HM Revenue & Customs

USA

http://www.irs.gov/

US Department of the Treasury, Internal Revenue Service

http://www.irs.gov/businesses/small/index.html

US Department of the Treasury, Internal Revenue Service
Small business and self-employed one-stop resource.

The mechanics of putting the practice together

4

Chapter contents

Location, location, location

Urban or countryside?

At first consideration urbanization offers people, but there is also a reasonable living to be made in the countryside, providing you are placed in an area that can support you economically.

So how do you know where to be? This is where your soon-to-be-acquired marketing skills will provide you with your answers.

Rural locations

Many practitioners seem to earn a good living in the countryside, but they do have to be in an area where potential patients have their own transport and an income that can pay for their services.

For a large proportion of people who live in a rural location, a visit to a local practitioner, who can save them a trip to the nearest city or local town, is very welcome.

Working in rural areas can create a rapid word-of-mouth referral system, but do bear in mind that bad news spreads more rapidly. Some practitioners like this very personal approach as they feel it helps them work more effectively and puts them in touch with the local community.

Working in an urban environment

In the city there will certainly be more buzz and the pace of life is much faster than in a rural location. Your patients may come from a much more diverse set of circumstances and each area of the city or town you locate yourself in will have a different character. Patients will arrive by a variety of transport, but this still is a factor you will have to take into account. Overheads may in some cases be higher in rentals and there will be more competition, but there will be a much larger market for potential patients.

Practitioners very often like to work in the two different environments as it gives them some variety.

One of the reasons you have trained in your particular field is to give you a lifestyle that you choose rather than your job dictating it for you. The choice of where you work is one of those aspects that has to be carefully considered.

General considerations

Generally speaking, the positioning of your clinic is one of the most important factors to take into consideration when starting up. If you are starting up from your own home this may be something you are not able to do much about. Certainly if your home is in a less than salubrious area your patients are likely to find this off-putting.

You may decide to deal with this problem by moving. The considerations for buying a new property must include at least a room you will be able to work out of. It may even be that you want to buy business premises that have accommodation attached.

Questions to ask regarding practice location

- *Is it on a thoroughfare?* The right signage will make potential patients aware of the clinic's presence. The downside is the possibility of noise, and business rates may be higher if they are assessed on numbers of people passing through.
- *Is there easy access?* Not all patients will come by car, so somewhere near a bus route or train station is useful. With respect to the Disability Discrimination Act 1995, access to premises has now become an issue and necessary alterations may be one of the costs you need to write into your business plan or take into consideration when looking at property to rent. If you are working from home you may want a separate patient access.
- *Is there good parking?* There is nothing more off-putting or stressful to patients than having to patrol the streets looking for somewhere to park their car before each visit, then being limited to the amount of time they can park.
- *Is the area a crime hotspot?* It should be easy if you do not have local knowledge to get this sort of information from the policeman assigned

as the neighbourhood constable. Small things such as fresh putty around the windows may indicate a break-in. Insurance companies do have a rating system for insuring properties in certain areas.

- *Is the security on the building adequate?* Locks and doors should be sturdy, and a burglar alarm is usually a good idea. You may also want to put locks on internal doors so that rooms can be locked while the practitioner is out, or to keep people from wandering around your home.
- *How much work will have to be done to the building to enable you to work from it?* There may be some internal decoration required but any major alterations will increase your starting costs. If you are renting, negotiate with the owner.
- *Is there planning for the intended usage?* The Local Authority is very unlikely to give planning permission retrospectively, particularly if there have been complaints from neighbouring properties.
- *How much are rates, electricity, and gas likely to be in a year?* This is useful information to gather, since it will be part of your budget. The previous incumbents or the owner should be able to give you an idea.

Business premises

The factors to consider become a little more complex.

- *Is the boiler safe and how new is it?* If you are renting, the boiler should have a landlord's certificate. If you are buying, you will need to know if the current boiler needs replacing.
- *Does the wiring of the building have a certificate?* This should be checked every 3 years to ensure the safety of the wiring.
- *Does the building conform to fire regulations?* Putting a clinic into a building may require alterations to the existing fire precautions. If it is not up to standard then you may invalidate your insurance.

If you are renting

- *What repairs or maintenance are you expected to perform?* Do not make the mistake of taking on a fully repairing lease where you are expected to repair the fabric of the building, or the expense could be exorbitant.
- *How long is the lease?* Are there any get-out clauses?

Renting a room

This simplifies matters greatly, as mostly you will be signing a contract that is in fact a licence. This should contain:

- Your name and the name of the person renting the room to you.
- The amount you pay to them and when you will pay it.

- When you will be using the room.
- What therapy you will be using.
- How much notice has to be given by either side to vacate the room.

Try to avoid exclusion clauses that prevent you working locally.

Be prepared to produce your qualifications and professional indemnity certificate. This is a reasonable request and one you should be making if the situation were reversed.

You in turn should check the following before you take a room:

- *Are there any other therapists of your discipline working from the premises?* If there are, how busy are they? There may be a possible conflict of interests. If you have been brought in because they are too busy to see any more patients then the association is likely to be a very productive one for you.
- *How many therapists of your discipline have there been on the premises and why did they leave?* A high turnover may indicate a problem with the clinic.
- *How are the bookings taken?* Is this something you do yourself or does the clinic do it for you? If they do take your bookings, do the people involved understand what you have to offer and will they take instructions from you as to what information needs to be passed on to patients?
- *How are practitioners allocated patients?* This can be very frustrating and costly if the patients likely to benefit the most from your service are not being directed to you.
- *Are they offering any other administrative services?* Will they ring patients for you? Chase up non-attendees? Take your money? Provide secretarial services?
- *What steps is the clinic taking to advertise your presence?*
- *Does the price you pay in rent reflect all the services available to you?*

Finally, ask:

- *Are they properly insured?* Ask to see their insurance certificates.
- *Is there public liability?* This should be on public display. You will be responsible for insuring your own equipment. Public liability and employee liability are generally included in your business insurance.
- *Is their equipment checked for safety at regular intervals?* You may well have a couch included in your fee. This requires a thorough maintenance check by someone who is qualified to certify it as safe.
- *Is the access suitable?* Does it comply with the Disability Discrimination Act?
- *How professional is the working environment?* What would your impression be if you were a potential patient? Cleanliness is very important and one of the best places to check this is by visiting the toilet and kitchen facilities. These should be well maintained and cared for.

How much space will I need?

If you are renting or buying premises do not guess at the space you will require. Draw it out on a plan. In its simplest form, squared graph paper is a cost-effective way of planning out your new business, but there are some relatively simple computer packages able to help you visualize your treatment room or clinic.

There is nothing worse than moving into your new clinic only to find you cannot move around the furniture. Look at the size of the furniture and the number of people who will be working there. Go down to an office equipment supplier and measure the sizes. In theory there should be 9.3 m^2 (100 square feet) per employee.

Large items can be bought lease purchase or lease hire. Try to find out what you have agreed to or you may end up paying for something which you may not necessarily own, and have to pay a minimal rent on it each year.

Office furniture

This can be bought second-hand, but do ensure that any upholstered items, such as chairs, are made of flame-retardant materials. This is signified by both a sticker on the item and a label attached by string, if the furniture is new. Otherwise the supplier you buy it from will have to certify in writing that the furniture is flame retardant.

Essential equipment

These are items that it would be impossible for most clinicians to manage without.

Answering machine

If you are not there or are unable to answer the phone, this will be the first port of call. It is worth investing the money in a good-quality machine, and probably one that also has a cordless phone facility, allowing you to answer the call regardless of where you are in your clinic.

If you have to use your home phone as the clinic phone, then the answering machine will be useful to screen calls you do not wish to take.

Couches

These can vary from lightweight and portable to heavy, static couches not intended for ease of mobility, but permanence.

Couches can be bought new or second-hand. New or reconditioned couches from a reputable supplier should come with a warranty. Those bought in a private sale should be checked carefully for cracks and worn areas. The couch will have to be safety checked once a year by a specialist who will be able to certify its safety. This will also be done for any other large pieces of equipment and electrical equipment that has to be plugged into the mains (see Ch. 8 on legislation). It is best not to buy second-hand, sight unseen.

It is interesting to note that when applying for a licence (in the case of acupuncturists and masseurs) that some local authorities are now asking what weight the couch can take. Do not assume that all your patients will be of an average size, and chiropractic and osteopathic couches particularly will receive a great deal of wear and tear in their working lifetime.

Computer equipment

It is possible to manage without this, but it is very useful, particularly for simple tasks such as word processing. Many professions such as homeopathy now have computerized repertorizing programs, which are of great help to the practitioner.

The Internet is now an important reference source, with many professional journals being accessible online. Emailing has become one of the fastest means of sending messages, although confidential information should be transmitted another way, by surface mail or fax. Many members of the professional associations have online discussion groups, which may be support for someone just starting up.

There are also hand-held computers, which contain word processing, spreadsheet, database and faxing facilities and are very reasonable in price. Some of the more basic ones, now being remanufactured under licence, can be very low cost and easier to carry around than a laptop.

Generally, there are two main suppliers of operating systems, Microsoft and Apple. Personal computers (PCs) usually run on Microsoft software, whereas the Apple operating system is integral to the Apple computer. A general PC tends to be easier to repair, although therapists who use Apple computers like their reliability.

You will only need the very latest computer if you want to create sophisticated graphics. Mostly you will need one capable of going on the Internet, and on which you can produce your letters, spreadsheet and databases. The important fact to be aware of is that it is easy to put a computer together, but for the uninitiated not all the components may be compatible.

Many computers are sold with a certain amount of software on them. If you are dealing with specialist suppliers, they can install this for you. Decide what you need and whether you are able to reduce the cost by buying and installing the software yourself. Installation of new software is now so simple that anyone can do it. The only problem may arise if for some reason the software is incompatible with your computer. If you are using specialists, you will be able to avoid this problem as you will have discussed your needs with them.

Do make sure you have the capability to back up data.

Do make sure that you have adequate antiviral, spyware and firewall programs if you use the Internet.

Photocopiers, scanners, faxes

These can be incorporated into one machine, which can be linked to a computer or used as a stand-alone device for photocopying or faxing. There is generally very little problem buying these from a large retailer, since if any problem occurs they can be easily exchanged.

If you are likely to be photocopying large amounts, then it is more economical to get a separate photocopier. If this is the case then it is better to hire, as the hire company is responsible for all the maintenance and repairs. Otherwise, providing the material you wish to photocopy is not confidential, then a high street printer will produce photocopies at a reasonable price.

The fax facility can be used on a separate line where it will be on automatic and permanently switched on. When starting out, however, this may prove expensive and it is possible to have the fax facility on the line used for voice and switch it on to receive only when required.

Consumer magazines may be useful to consult to see where the best buys are for computer equipment.

X-ray equipment

This is a substantial piece of equipment to buy and usually beyond the budget for a new chiropractor.

In many cases it may be worth looking for a clinic or hospital that can perform an X-ray series for you. It may take 2 weeks to generate a report through the NHS, but the patient may have had the problem for some time. If you do suspect patients of having a serious condition worth X-raying, then it is likely anyway that you will pass them straight on to their GP.

Basic information about X-ray equipment is included here as a way of informing a practitioner of the cost and complexity of having a unit in a clinic.

New equipment, which will have to be fitted professionally, may cost over £20 000, and probably half that amount if it is reconditioned.

A radiation protection advisor will have to be consulted as to what measures to take to ensure safety. This is likely to require some building work, possibly including lead shielding of some kind.

Film processing is now done with machines whose results are consistent, providing they are cleaned and the developing and fixing fluids are kept fresh. The machine, like the X-ray equipment, has to be serviced once a year.

A reputable company will not fit a processor into a room unless it has the following:

- Good ventilation with an extractor fan.
- A sink.
- A water supply with the correct fittings to hook the processor up to.

The room should be used specifically for the purpose of producing X-ray films and nothing else. If the room is not light-tight, then a light-tight facility must be bought that attached to the processor to allow you to change the film.

A radiation protection advisor, usually appointed by your professional association, will be making regular visits to ensure you are producing films of a suitable quality and that your facilities meet acceptable standards.

In addition you will need:

- X-ray cassettes.
- Films.
- Light-tight box to store films in.
- Gonad shielding.
- Filters.
- Radiation exposure badges – one for each person using the facility.
- Light marker for marking films with patient details.
- Fixer and developer.

The local health and safety officer will also have to be informed you are using an X-ray unit.

Additional costs should include the servicing fees, which are expensive as the engineers are specialists and you pay for their time from the minute they leave home to the minute they get back. Your radiation protection advisor is also an expensive item.

Taking all this into account makes it very obvious that an X-ray facility is not for the faint hearted, not only in terms of expense but in the expenditure of time required to maintain it correctly and ensure your staff's health.

Tax related to equipment

When you buy equipment you will need to keep the details safe, as the HM Revenue and Customs may want to know:

- What was purchased.
- When it was purchased.
- How much it cost.
- What percentage was used for the business.

If you sell it they will want to know:

- What was sold.
- When it was sold.
- How much money you made from the sale or whether there was a part-exchange – this might occur in the case of a car.

Keep all the records for your accountant.

Hiring equipment

Commonly, this tends to be items like photocopiers or static hydraulic couches which are necessary in large-volume practices. Occasionally, however, other types of equipment may be necessary, and it may be preferable to hire rather than making an expensive purchase you cannot afford.

Points to consider

- *Insurance.* Who is responsible for insuring it?
- *Minimum hire period.*
- *Where is the equipment to be kept?* The hire company has the right to insist that the equipment you hire from them is kept in one place. You may be allowed to move it around, providing you notify them. If it is portable and you need to take it with you, check to see if this is all right. They may also want to be assured that it is being kept in the appropriate conditions with suitable security.
- *Who is allowed to use it?* Does the contract specify this?
- *Early termination of contract.* There may be a minimum period of time for which you were signed up to hire the equipment. If you wish to relieve yourself of it early you may still be liable to pay the remaining payments or there may be some type of penalty clause. Look to see what the arrangements are for termination of the contract.
- *Service or maintenance.* You need to know, if the piece of equipment becomes faulty in any way, that the hire company will repair or replace it as quickly as possible. Ensure also that they are responsible for the maintenance checks, particularly the electrical check.
- *Your obligations.* You must ensure that the best care is taken of the equipment you hire, as you will be liable for replacing it if it is lost, or repairing it if it is broken. You must also ensure that the rental payments are paid on time. If you are the forgetful type or find this a chore, a direct debit may be helpful.
- *The obligations of the hire company.* They must supply you with your equipment in good order, as it must be safe to use and fit for purpose. Check the equipment thoroughly before you use it. They should let you use the equipment, without interference, providing you are looking after it and your payments are up to date.

You must always check the terms and conditions of any contract *before* you sign it. There may be hidden costs in the small print that may not be appreciated on a cursory glance.

Hire purchase

This is a type of hiring contract, with a view to eventually owning the piece of equipment, or a car. You pay an initial deposit or payment, after which come further regular instalments which will cover the purchase price. Within these payments will be an interest charge. The final payment is usually not part of the hire but an '*option to buy*'.

This is where you must *check the contract carefully* to see whether you have been sold this option or whether you will merely continue to lease the equipment for as long as you want it at a minimal charge. If you are not careful, you will have paid a great deal of money for something you will not ultimately own.

The sellers' obligations

They are obliged to present the equipment to you in good, safe and workable condition as soon as they have received the first payment from you.

They should let you use the equipment, without interference, providing you are looking after it and you keep up the payments.

Your obligations

You must look after the equipment for the period of the hire purchase agreement. Once you have made the final payment, the equipment is yours.

Backing out of a hire purchase agreement

If you do have problems keeping up repayments there is usually a clause in the contract to cover this. Quite often, you will only be able to back out of an agreement after a certain number of payments have been made or amount of time has elapsed since the start of the agreement.

Once you have returned the item there should be no more to pay.

If you owe money to the seller when you decide to terminate the agreement then you will be liable for the outstanding amounts up to the date of the termination.

Check the agreement as they all vary.

Stock

This is an issue for practitioners such as herbalists and homeopaths. Consider whether it may be more cost-effective to use a prescription service in the case of homeopathic remedies or loose herbs.

It is certainly very expensive to set up a herbal pharmacy, although some companies offer credit or a special start-up deal for new practitioners. It may also be difficult due to lack of space to store herbs and, if you work from more than one premises, expensive to stock all of them.

Services

Water

Even a relatively large clinic only uses as much water as domestic use. Check the tariff on the building, as sometimes the business rates which are in place are more relevant to a large factory than your clinic. If the rate is unmetered, the cost can be alarmingly high purely because you are in a business premises. Before you even sign the contract get the building metered as part of the rental or purchase agreement.

Electricity

Make sure you read the meter as soon as you take over and notify the electricity board.

Check the meter readings, although with business a meter reader usually visits before the quarterly bill.

Gas

Again, check the reading. It will also be worth taking out an insurance policy with your supplier or a reputable firm. Parts may be not be included in the policy, but this is a reasonable fee considering the cost of calling out heating engineers and paying for their time. They will be obliged to attend your call as quickly as possible and the service will also ensure that your boiler is safe.

Telephone

It is a good idea to have a mobile as well as a landline phone, particularly when you are setting up.

Landline

There are an overwhelming number of options. Ask around and see what experience people you know have had from different providers. As with any service, the after-sales service is all important. Your time is valuable and you do not want to waste an hour of it waiting on a phone to speak to someone.

Not only do you need to consider putting in the line, but also the type of service you get with it. You may want to use voicemail, divert, call waiting and numerous other services.

You need to have provision for rapid repair, in case there is a fault. It is possible to divert the calls to another line or a mobile but repairs under a normal system may take a period of days. Although it has to be said that if the phone company is at fault, they will cover the cost of the calls to the mobile, it may cause logistical problems.

You may therefore want to buy an insurance package, particularly if you have a clinic that has a small exchange with extensions, as the telephone company may charge to send an engineer to repair the internal system. An insurance package also assures you that they have to start repairs within a few hours of your call and your repair will be prioritized.

You cannot afford loss of earning just because you will not spend a little extra.

You may require more than one phone line in to the premises for several reasons:

- The ability to leave a fax on automatic.
- To have a separate line on a withheld number for practitioners in the clinic to make calls without blocking incoming calls from potential patients.

- If you decide to have a security system that communicates with a central monitoring station, this will require a clean phone line free of fax or modem interference.

Mobile

This is an extra expense, but as many of your competitors will have this facility, you cannot afford to be without it.

It will give you enormous flexibility as to where and when you can take calls. If the clinic is not busy initially, you can have your calls diverted to the mobile so that no matter where you are you can receive calls. There is nothing worse than picking up your answering machine messages only to find that potential patients have booked in elsewhere or just not left a message because they will not talk to an answering machine.

A mobile phone may also be a lifeline for patients if the clinic is closed and a brief conversation is all that is required to reassure them.

Caller ID is now standard on mobile phones, which will allow you to see where calls are being made from. Some practitioners refuse to answers calls with no assigned number on the principle that they are sales or nuisance calls and a genuine patient will leave a message.

Security

If you are renting a room this may not be an issue that bothers you, particularly if you remove your equipment, but if the premises are damaged and have to be closed for repairs you may lose business.

If you rent or buy whole premises this will be an issue for you, since the property will be unattended when the clinic is closed.

When working from home, serious consideration should be given to security, since you will have to tell your patients when you are going away.

If you have expensive equipment on your premises it would be a false economy not to have a system that is monitored. The package should also include priority repair of the landline if it is damaged or deliberately cut. The longer the phone system is down the more vulnerable you become.

If a security system is in place and is monitored, then the firm you use will have to have a list of keyholders with their numbers, just in case you are not available.

If you are responsible for the building you will have to make allowances for an alarm reset charge, out-of-hours boarding, renewal of glass and repair of any damage done. Although costs can be recovered on your insurance policy, there will be an excess to pay. Too many claims made in one year may make it difficult to renew your insurance as you will be classed as a liability, or push up the cost of your insurance, so you will have to make a judgement as to whether you cover the cost yourself.

Monitored systems cannot be used on a telephone line that uses a fax machine or modem, as the signal may trigger the alarm at the central monitoring centre. This will also mean paying for another telephone line to be installed. The line used for voice can be used for the system, but you will hear, at intervals, a low beeping for a few seconds as the carrier signal passes down the line.

Fire

Regulations will be covered in more detail in Chapter 8 on legislation, but you will need to know what extinguishers and signage you need, so that this can be added to the costs.

Financial checklist so far

Equipment

Answering machine

Couch
- Couch cover
- Pillows

Computer

- Software
- Security software

Fax, scanner photocopier – buy separately or together

Diagnostic equipment

This may have already been bought as part of your course.

Stethoscope
Otoscope
Auriculoscope
Tuning forks

Furniture

Desk
Chairs

Consumables

Head rolls
Couch rolls
Soap, etc.

Decoration

Flooring
Paint and/or wallpaper
Pictures

Car

Cost to buy
Insurance
Repairs

Utilities

Gas
Electricity
Water
Telephone

Any items that are usually considered household goods such as kettles and vacuum cleaners may not be covered by certain guarantees. Do check before buying.

Dealing with professionals in the start-up and running of your practice

5

Chapter contents

Research resources

Before you even start to make contact with the people who will be directly involved in the various elements of your business, do not forget the public sector facilities that are free and easily available for reference. These valuable resources are certainly vital for the research you will need to do to establish your practice within your community.

Public libraries

Larger libraries in towns and cities may have a business library which will contain much of the information you will need, to find not only professional services but also general information on starting businesses.

Most urban libraries now have an online catalogue system, which allows you to perform a search from the comfort of your own home. You will be able to see if a book you are looking for is in the library or on loan and, if you have a library ticket, reserve a book or extend the loan of books you have borrowed. You may also be able to request certain books that are not in your library, although a nominal charge will be levied for this service.

Having a library ticket will also give you online access to the EBSCO system, which will allow you to read many journals and newspapers free and online. Local newspapers are often made available this way, which will provide you with useful information about your local community.

Public library staff are usually very enthusiastic and helpful and generally enjoy the challenge of finding answers for the library's members.

If for some reason you do not have access to the Internet at home, the library offers a free Internet service. Providing you produce a valid library ticket, you will be able to book time on one of the library's computers.

The Citizens' Advice Bureau (CAB)

The Citizens' Advice Bureau may be the first port of call for many people who need basic advice on money matters, but it is also able to advise on many queries. It is a nationwide organization, largely run by trained volunteers who can offer advice, and has been operating since 1939. The advice offered is free, impartial, independent and confidential and may point you in the right direction to find the information you need.

No CAB will recommend commercial suppliers or trades, but they do keep a directory of local law firms, which will allow you to find out how much experience each firm has and the areas in which they specialize.

If you meet with a financial or legal problem and you are not sure whether you need to resort to professional help, the CAB may be the place to go.

The major problems that the CAB deals with are financial difficulties, and they are often able to negotiate with creditors on the client's behalf or give management plans to help people get out of debt. Hopefully you will not find this service necessary but it is useful to know that this facility is there.

Do not forget that although the volunteers are trained, they are not usually qualified lawyers or accountants, but they will provide the best service they can.

The Internet

This is a valuable tool for research that it is possible to use from the comfort of your own home. It will enable you to examine the websites of the relevant organizations and governing bodies. This should give you a better idea of the stringency with which their members are vetted and whether there is a method of quality assurance. Very often there will be a facility to check for members near you.

Specialist advice and skills

The most common way of choosing people whose specialist services you will require is by personal recommendations from people who have had positive experiences of them. Their credibility is further enhanced by membership of a recognized professional association. This is by no means foolproof but these precautions should help to ensure several things:

- That any work undertaken will be of the highest quality.
- That if they are working on your premises, they will be insured against personal injury and professional negligence.
- That, if there is a problem at a later stage, you will be able to lodge a complaint that should be properly investigated.

Never take on anyone's services just because they are a friend or relative, without checking the quality of their work.

Solicitors

You will at some point have to consult with a solicitor. Usually this is for contracts of one form or another, or to check on various legal points. If you are unfortunate enough to be involved in a problem such as a breach of contract or an accident at work, then it is likely you will need a solicitor to untangle the complex web of legal issues.

Legislation is constantly changing and a solicitor will be your means to ensure that you are up to date with all legal requirements in the running of your business.

All solicitors in private practice must hold a practising certificate issued by the Law Society. This ensures that you are seeing someone who is properly qualified and insured.

A small firm may appear to give a more personal service, but a large firm will have specialist departments, commercial law being one of them.

The first meeting

The Law Society has a very informative website regarding approaching and interacting with a solicitor. Solicitors will usually charge for their time; therefore it is important that you use your time with them efficiently. Below are salient facts extracted from the Law Society website (see p. 53):

Before the meeting

- Make sure you have all your questions written down and all the paperwork you need together to take with you.
- As a point of etiquette do let the solicitor know if you are bringing someone with you. This may be because you need a specific person to be there, for instance your accountant, or someone for general reassurance. Meeting a solicitor for the first time can be a daunting experience.
- You might also want to check how long the meeting will be so you can be sure you will cover all the important points in the meeting.

At the meeting

- Do arrive promptly, since the solicitor will have other clients after you and it is not desirable to be charged for time you did not use because you were late.

- Make notes, since an event or conversation that appeared clear at the time might seem less clear later on, or you may forget something.
- Be brief and accurate in answering your solicitor's questions.
- Show the solicitor all the relevant documents you have brought with you.
- Ask for a written summary of the advice you have been given.

You should be able to ask about charges before you consult with your solicitor, so that you will have an idea of the amount you will have to budget for. Do not forget that paperwork generated and phone calls may also incur a charge.

It is quite acceptable to investigate charges that are likely to be levied by different solicitors. Some solicitors will charge a nominal fee or make no charge at all for an orientation interview.

Lawyer for Your Business is a network of solicitors' firms around the country who offer free half-hour consultations. This may be useful if you are not sure of your requirements. Contacting the Law Society by email on lfyb@lawsociety.org.uk will enable to you to ascertain if there is a Lawyer for Your Business solicitor near you.

Accountancy

It is not necessary to have an accountant, but with the complexities of legislation and tax even the smallest business would be wise to use the services of one.

A good accountant will:

- Endeavour to keep your tax bills down legitimately.
- Advise you on the most cost-effective ways of running your business
- Prepare your end-of-year accounts.
- Give you advice on how he thinks your business is performing and what adjustments you may have to make.

One of the major professional bodies for accountants is the Institute of Chartered Accountants in England and Wales, while the equivalent body north of the border is the Institute of Chartered Accountants in Scotland. The Association of Chartered Certified Accountants (ACCA) is a large international accountancy body. All members of these associations must follow a code of conduct and are expected to meet the associations' standards of professionalism. They also hold professional indemnity insurance.

Architects

Generally speaking, minor internal changes to a building do not require planning permission.

If you are undertaking serious alterations, changing the internal structure of a listed building or extending it, then it is a very good idea to employ the services of an architect who is used to dealing with the building regulations and the processes involving the local authority planning office. Unless you are very experienced in this area and have a great deal of spare time, it is not cost-effective for you to personally manage this type of project.

Qualified architects are registered with the Architects Registration Board (ARB).

Remember that providing they can work safely, the builders you contract to do your work will get on with the job as directed by you. It is not their job to check whether you have planning permission.

Financial services and insurance

Any bona fide insurance broker or consultant should be a member of the Financial Services Authority (FSA). The FSA now monitors every aspect of the insurance industry and, as with the professional bodies for solicitors and accountants, has a code of conduct that is rigorously applied.

A financial advisor will assist you in making investment, pension, mortgage, life insurance and permanent healthcare decisions. You are paying for him to search for the best deal he can get you. This may be based more on financial considerations than the actual products, so as well as looking at prices your financial advisor should also be looking for something that fits your specifications. Make this clear when talking to him.

There is nothing to stop you ringing around yourself, but it will take time and some effort to understand and negotiate a suitable deal. There are now also many online facilities that will perform a search based on your requirements.

You may well receive information on a new policy each year. Check to see it is comparable with the last one you had, and compare the price. There may be some form filling required each time but the savings involved may be worth it.

Some brokers who issue professional liability insurance, may also be general insurers and are well situated to understand the sometimes complex needs of general insurance matters of the complementary field.

Skilled craftsmen

Always get a written quotation from whomever you are dealing with and shop around for the best deal. Cheapest is not necessarily the best. It is a good idea to view the work of a person you are potentially hiring if the work you are asking them to do is substantial. Usually word of mouth referral can be helpful, but there are various professional associations that should enable you to select someone competent.

Computer services

Computers can be bought new or reconditioned. As with most electrical equipment they are generally better bought new. The expensive part of the system will be the central processing unit (CPU), which is the heart of the system, and where most of the money is best spent.

The other parts such as the monitor and the keyboard do not need to be state of the art and can be acquired relatively cheaply and without any high degree of technical knowledge. A high-quality screen may be essential if eyestrain or visual impairment is a factor to be considered.

Large computer retail outlets have good offers for initial purchase, but their after-sales service may not be adequate. Computer specifications may also be limited. Sometimes it is better to go for a small independent firm, which can produce a computer to suit your needs. Although they may be slightly more expensive, the after-sales service is likely to be more personal, easy to contact and quickly able to solve your problems, probably on the same day.

There are several qualifications available to computer specialists, ranging from National Vocational Qualifications (NVQs) to university degrees. Microsoft also runs accreditation courses. Obviously, the depth of knowledge is likely to vary greatly between specialists. A careful examination of *Yellow Pages* and websites may help to narrow down the field. A good website is a must for the computer industry. The organization and presentation of the website may give an indication of their professionalism. There may also be a list of firms they supply. See if there are any names you can recognize. Reputable firms will only tolerate good workmanship.

The local Chamber of Commerce will have a list of members in this field. Generally speaking they will only join if they are serious about their business. Even if you are not a member of the Chamber of Commerce you may be able to attend some functions, enabling you to meet potential contacts.

Generally, a good-quality specialist computer firm does not differentiate in their enthusiasm for conducting business between a single domestic user and a large company wanting sophisticated multi-unit computers.

It is also important when choosing a firm to seek one that can give you constant cover, even if someone goes on holiday or is ill. This can often be a problem with a one-man business. Make sure that there is someone available for cover, or choose a slightly larger firm so that there will always be someone to help you if there is a problem.

Unfortunately, as yet, there is no governing body for this particular area and anyone can claim to perform the task for you. Personal recommendation still seems to be the most reliable way to choose a supplier.

Plumbers

The Institute of Plumbing and Heating Engineering (IPHE) or the Institute of Plumbing (IP), (which is basically the same organization) is the professional body for the UK plumbing and heating industry. Members range from sole proprietors to engineers in industry.

If you require a plumber who is able install or maintain a boiler, then your will need someone who is CORGI registered. Engineers should carry a card to identify exactly what work they are competent to carry out. There is also an expiry date on the card so you will be able to see whether they have a current certificate.

The CORGI website also contains helpful information on gas and the law (see p. 54).

Electricians

The competence of any member of the Electrical Contractors' Association (ECA) is overseen by the Building Research Establishment (BRE) certification scheme.

Looking through the ECA website (see p. 54) will tell you what the electrical contractor performing your work is eligible to undertake. This includes general electrical wiring and security and fire alarm installation.

Fire

If you are renting or buying commercial premises, you may well find, if you have applied for planning permission, that you will receive a visit from a representative of the local fire brigade. Look upon this as a useful exercise and helpful free advice from someone well qualified in fire safety assessment who will be able to give impartial advice on whether or not your equipment, signage, fire exits, etc. are in compliance with fire regulations. You should check on this anyway if you are working from commercial premises.

Becoming compliant may require nothing more complicated than a few of the right fire extinguishers, but it may involve installation of sprinkler systems and provision of emergency exits.

There are specialist firms who will advise you free of charge in anticipation of your buying their equipment and signage.

It is wise to ensure, whatever the circumstances, that the new premises you are taking over meet safety requirements. Non-compliance may mean a fine, or even worse a loss of life.

Firms who are members of associations such as the National Security Inspectorate (NSI) or the British Fire Protection Systems Association (BFPSA) will be able to conduct a fire risk assessment and supply the correct equipment. Your premises will be thoroughly inspected every 6 months to ensure that they meet the current standards. They will be able to issue you with a Certificate of Compliance for the systems you have installed, which at a simple level will be smoke detectors and the appropriate fire extinguishers.

Security

The National Security Inspectorate (NSI) also provides inspection services for the security industry. The Security Systems and Alarms Inspection Board (SSAIB) is another regulatory body.

Members of the Electrical Contractors' Association (ECA) may well be certified to install fire detection as well as security equipment.

Builders

Generally speaking, a builder who is a member of the Federation of Master Builders must meet a standard set of criteria and the Federation will investigate any complaints made.

Joiners

Very often if you are having work done by a builder, the joiner will come as part of the package. If you do hire an individual carpenter and do not have a recommendation, it is worth looking for a member from the Institute of Carpenters, the Guild of Master Craftsmen or the British Woodworking Federation.

Conclusion

There is no definitive way to find the correct person to perform the job or function that you require them for. Membership of an association or recognized body does ensure that you are dealing with someone who is properly qualified, and who is insured. You are also more likely to be able to seek recourse for any work that is unacceptable.

Although verbal agreements are contracts, they are not tangible and therefore difficult to prove if there is a dispute. It is important to have anything agreed in writing.

Faxing orders or letters is efficient and simple and gives you a date and time on your fax report. If an order is complicated or there may be a misinterpretation of what you have said, the fax will clarify the matter and act as a written record.

If a letter or document is particularly important, make sure it has to be signed for at the other end and its progress in the postal system can be monitored. This way, the party you are dealing with is unable to say that it has not been received. If you merely wish to prove that you have sent something, ask for a certificate of posting at the post office.

Useful websites

Australia

Solicitors

http://www.lawaccess.nsw.gov.au/

Law Access Online
Legal information and advice services. Government site. New South Wales.

http://www.lawcouncil.asn.au/about.html

The Law Council of Australia

Accountants

http://www.cpaaustralia.com.au/cps/rde/xchg

Certified Public Accountants Australia

http://www.icaa.org.au/
Institute of Chartered Accountants Australia

Architects
http://www.architecture.com.au/
Royal Australian Institute of Architects

Financial services and insurance
http://www.apra.gov.au/
Australian Prudential Regulation Authority (APRA)

Plumbers
http://www.heating.com.au/
Master Plumbers' and Mechanical Services Association of Australia

http://www.plumber.com.au/
Master Plumbers' and Mechanical Services Association of Australia

Electricians
http://www.neca.asn.au/
National Electrical and Communications Association (NECA)

Fire
http://www.fpaa.com.au/
Fire Protection Association Australia

Security
http://www.neca.asn.au/
National Electrical and Communications Association (NECA)

Builders
http://www.aib.org.au/
Australian Institute of Building

Joiners
It has not been possible to find these but they may be part of the Australian Institute of Building.

Canada

Many websites are bilingual.

Solicitors

http://www.bbb.org/

Better Business Bureau
Allows you to check if there have been any consumer issues with a business you intend using. Companies who are registered with them will carry their logo on their advertising.

http://www.cba.org/CBA/Gate.asp

Canadian Bar Association

http://www.communitylegal.mb.ca/

Community Legal Education Association
This is a charity organization providing Manitobans with legal information.

http://www.flsc.ca/

Federation of Law Societies of Canada
National Coordinating body for all 14 law societies in Canada.

Accountants

http://www.cica.ca/index.cfm/ci_id/17150/la_id/1.htm

Institute of Chartered Accountants

http://www.cga-online.org/servlet/custom/workspace

Association of Certified General Accountants

http://www.cma-canada.org/index.cfm/ci_id/45/la_id/1.htm

Certified Management Accountants

Architects

http://www.oaa.on.ca/

Ontario Association of Architects

http://www.raic.org/

Royal Architectural Institute of Canada
French and English languages.

Financial services and insurance

http://www.cfp-ca.org/public/public_industrydir.asp

Financial Planners Standards Council
Provides information on what to look for in a financial planner and a search engine to find you nearest financial planner.

http://www.clhia.ca/index_en.htm

Canadian Life and Health Insurance Association

http://www.ibc.ca/home.asp

Insurance Bureau of Canada

http://www.osfi-bsif.gc.ca/

Office of the Superintendent of Financial Instructions of Canada
Governmental body implementing legislation in the insurance company generally.

Tradesmen

http://www.bbb.org/

Better Business Bureau
Allows you to check if there have been any consumer issues with a business you intend using.

Plumbers

http://www.phccweb.org/

Plumbing Heating and Cooling Contractors Association
National Association.

http://www.ua.org/

United Association of Journeymen Apprentices of the Plumbing and Pipe Fitting Industry of the United States and Canada

Electricians

http://www.ceca.org/english/index.html

Canadian Electrical Contractors Association

Security

http://www.canasa.org/

Canadian Security Association

http://www.ulc.ca/consumer/

Underwriters' Laboratories of Canada

Fire

http://www.nfpa.org/

National Fire Protection Association

New Zealand

Governmental websites are bilingual.

Lawyers
http://www.nz-lawsoc.org.nz/
New Zealand Law Society

Accountants
http://newzealand.accaglobal.com/
Association of Certified Chartered Accountants.

http://www.nzica.com/
Institute of Chartered Accountants New Zealand

Architects
http://www.nzia.co.nz/
New Zealand Institute of Architects

Financial services and insurance
http://www.fpia.org.nz/
Financial Planners and Insurance Advisors Association

Plumbers
http://www.pgdb.co.nz/index.php?sh=01&h2=01
Master Plumbers, Gasfitters and Drainlayers NZ
This is a governmentally appointed body that promotes high standards in the industry of work, professional conduct and the protection of public health and safety through the registration and licensing of competent plumbers, gasfitters and drainlayers.

Electricians
http://www.ecanz.org.nz/
Electrical Contractors Association of New Zealand (ECANZ)

Fire and security
http://www.fireprotection.org.nz/
New Zealand Fire Protection Association
Some contractors are also electricians and also deal with security.

Builders
http://www.bcito.org.nz/
Building and Construction Industry Training Organisation
This organization is appointed by the Government to develop and implement qualifications in various aspects of the building and construction sector, therefore setting an expected standard for tradesmen.

http://www.certified.co.nz/

Certified Builders Association of New Zealand

http://www.masterbuilder.org.nz/

Master Builders Association

Joiners

http://www.jito.org.nz/

Joinery Industry Training Organisation

This organization organizes training and sets standards for tradesmen in the joinery industry.

UK

http://www.adviceguide.org.uk/

Citizens' Advice Bureau

Solicitors

http://www.lawsociety.org.uk/home.law

The Law Society

Accountants

http://www.acca.co.uk

Association of Chartered Certified Accountants

http://www.icaew.co.uk

Institute of Chartered Accountants in England and Wales

http://www.icas.org.uk

Institute of Chartered Accountants in Scotland

Architects

http://www.arb.org.uk/

Architects Registration Board

Financial services and insurance

http://www.fsa.gov.uk/

Financial Services Authority

Plumbers and heating engineers

http://iphe.org.uk

Institute of Plumbing and Heating Engineering

http://www.corgi-gas-safety.com/
Confederation for Registration of Gas Installers (CORGI)

Electricians
http://www.brecertification.co.uk/
Building Research Establishment (BRE)

http://www.eca.co.uk/
Electrical Contractors' Association (ECA)

Fire and security
http://www.bfpsa.org.uk/
British Fire Protection Systems Association (BFPSA)

http://www.fireservice.co.uk/
Fire service

http://www.nsi.org.uk/
National Security Inspectorate (NSI)

http://www.ssaib.co.uk/
Security Systems and Alarms Inspection Board (SSAIB)

Builders
http://www.builders.org.uk/nfb/
Federation of Master Builders

Joiners
http://www.bwf.org.uk/
British Woodworking Federation

http://www.carpenters-institute.org/
Institute of Carpenters

http://www.thegmcgroup.com/theguild/index.html
Guild of Master Craftsmen

USA

Solicitors
http://icdr.sullivan.edu/
International Center for Dispute Resolution
This is a resource website for resolving disputes.

Lawyers

http://www.abanet.org/about/home.html

American Bar Association

http://www.abanet.org/barserv/stlobar.html

American Bar Association State and Local Bar Association Directory

http://www.business.gov/topics/business_laws/hiring_lawyer/index.html

Business.gov
Website on hiring a lawyer.

Accountants

http://www.aicpa.org/index.htm

American Institute of Certified Public Accountants

Architects

http://www.aia.org/

American Institute of Architects

http://www.sara-national.org/

Society of American Registered Architects

Financial services and insurance

http://www.aicpcu.org/

American Institute for Chartered Property Casualty Underwriters and the Insurance Institute of America

http://www.cfp-board.org/

Certified Financial Planner

http://www.fpanet.org/

Financial Planning Association

http://www.naic.org/index.htm

National Association of Insurance Commissioners
These are insurance regulators and cover all the states. Database available on insurers.

Tradesmen

http://www.bbb.org/

Better Business Bureau
Allows you to check if there have been any consumer issues with a business you intend using. Companies who are registered with them will carry their logo on their advertising.

Construction

http://contractors-license.org/

Construction contractors, electricians and plumbers should all be licensed by the relevant state. This website enables you to check if they have a licence.

Plumbers

http://www.aspe.org/

American Society of Plumbing Engineers

http://www.ua.org/

United Association of Journeymen Apprentices of the Plumbing and Pipe Fitting Industry of the United States and Canada

Heating and air-conditioning

http://www.acca.org/

Air Conditioning Contractors of America

http://www.ashrae.org/

American Society of Heating Refrigerating and Air Conditioning Engineers

Electricians

http://www.alarm.org/

National Burglar and Fire Alarm Association

http://www.necanet.org/

National Electrical Contractors Association

Fire

http://www.nfpa.org/

National Fire Protection Association

Builders

http://www.nari.org/

National Association of the Remodelling Industry
This can include builders, electricians, etc.

Insurance 6

Chapter contents

Insurance is an item you cannot afford to ignore, particularly when starting your own business. Being self-employed may or may not affect all your current policies such as household, car and life. For example, if you operate a mobile practice then your car insurance may be affected.

Types of insurance

There are several types of insurance that you may need.

Professional indemnity

Professional indemnity is usually a requirement of membership of a professional body. You should not work without this type of cover even if you do not belong to a professional body, in case a patient wishes to conduct a claim against you for injury or damage as a result of the treatment you carried out.

If you do not wish to belong to a professional body, then some insurance companies will insure you as a properly qualified complementary therapist, providing you are able to supply the appropriate certificates.

Public liability

Public liability cover is used if a member of the public, a patient, or someone visiting the premises has been injured on your property. It is not compulsory, but is something that you should take out. Your business insurance will usually provide this type of cover for you as a matter of course even if the centre you work in has public liability insurance.

The people you are renting the room from should also have public liability insurance. If they do not, then question whether it is wise to work there.

If you are working from home, then as well as checking to see if your household insurance needs changing, you should also check the terms of your mortgage as this may also be affected.

Employer's liability

This is issued along with the business insurance whether you have employees or not, and by law should be retained for 40 years. It will cover you should any member of staff have an accident on the premises and try to prove that the accident came about as a result of your negligence.

Employer's liability will also cover for such items as theft by employees and assault on employees while engaged in the duty of taking money to the bank. Do check that any temporary staff are adequately covered in the terms of your insurance.

Dispensing insurance

It is now necessary to be covered for any herbal formulations or loose remedies of any kind that are made up on site at the clinic and dispensed by someone other than the practitioner. This employee should be adequately trained to perform this task.

This type of cover is usually available as an addition to your existing professional indemnity cover.

Product liability

Your professional indemnity should provide you with cover for anything you might sell, which might be anything from homeopathic and herbal remedies to pillows.

If a patient has reacted to a product in some way that was unforeseen or patients have injured themselves and the issue is not one of professional negligence, then the product liability cover will come into action. Generally if the item is sold sealed, with the seal unbroken, and is faulty in some way, the case would be taken up with the manufacturer or wholesaler.

Practitioner culpability only comes into this scenario if there has been negligence in diagnosis and use of herbs and there has been a problem. If there is no evidence of professional negligence, but there is a problem with the herbs and they have been supplied by a prescription service, the following should apply:

- If the wrong herbs have been dispensed, the prescription service should be liable.
- If the prescription service has supplied poor-quality herbs that have caused a problem, the prescription service should again be liable.

Some professional associations provide a list of approved suppliers to avoid this problem occurring and you may find you are not insured if you do not use a recognized supplier.

Business interruption

If anything serious affects the place in which you work, for example flooding, and customers could go elsewhere while you are sorting out the problem, and might not return, insurance for this eventuality is important.

Some policies will help by providing funds for alternative accommodation if the problem can take more than a few weeks to resolve.

Buildings insurance

Contents

This will cover equipment and furniture. In other words all the parts of your clinic that are not part of the structure of the building.

Stock

This will include saleable items such as herbs, remedies, pillows, etc.

General notes

Insurance should cover fire and flood and theft. It is probably a very good idea before renting or buying premises to ensure that they are in an area that is not prone to flooding, as this may not be covered under the terms of your insurance.

You are under an obligation to disclose anything that may affect the underwriter or the policy terms, even if it is adverse. Failing to do this, either as a mistake, omission or misrepresentation, may invalidate the policy, leaving you to foot the bill for whatever misfortune has occurred.

If you have a large claim, the insurance company may well send a loss adjuster to see to what extent the claim is valid. Make sure that the value of replacing your equipment is kept up to date; there is nothing worse than finding you are under-insured.

Permanent healthcare insurance

This is very important in case injury or serious illness prevents you working, particularly if you have a family to support. It should provide you with some level of income if you are ill or have an accident, but it does not cover all your income, only a part of it.

Policies vary widely as to when they start paying out. The more expensive the policy the sooner you receive payments. Most do not start for 4–6 weeks.

Private healthcare

You will be self-employed and the only way to earn money is if you are physically working in your clinic. This means you cannot afford to be ill for too long. This insurance will mean you receive treatment more quickly than you might otherwise do under the NHS.

Vehicle insurance

It is compulsory to carry motor vehicle insurance and you must insure your legal liability for injury to others and damage to their property arising from the use of your vehicle on the road – third party insurance.

Third-party cover is compulsory but may be a false economy, considering the amount you may have to pay out in the case of an accident. Fully comprehensive cover, though more expensive, will give peace of mind.

If you intend using your car in mobile treatment work then you must inform your insurance company or your insurance may be invalidated.

Legal

There is a possibility that you may face a legal action, which may come from a disgruntled employee claiming unfair dismissal. It does come at extra expense, but it may be worth covering any legal costs.

Where do you get insurance?

Occasionally, some professional indemnity brokers will also be able to advise on other insurance policies. This can be helpful since they should have a good understanding of your particular needs.

Another option is to use general brokers. Their job should be to find you the best deal for a reasonable sum of money. Brokers generally work on commission, which will be paid to them from the insurance companies once a new client has been engaged. It is therefore important to tell them exactly what your requirements are so that they can get you the best deal possible.

The advantage of having a broker is that if there is a problem with your insurance claim she will be able to act under your instruction as an informed intermediary between you and the insurance company. The Financial Services Authority should be able to put you in contact with a reputable broker, who will be able to discuss your needs and explain the different types of insurance you might need.

There is nothing to stop you ringing round yourself to find a policy, and the Internet now has many sites that allow you to look for a policy by filling out online forms.

Do check how much the excess of each policy is and see if the saving made on the policy due to a large excess is a worthwhile saving long term.

Do remember you are paying for the service.

You should receive information on a new policy each year. Check to see that its coverage is comparable with the last one you had, and compare the price. It is tedious to start again but may be worth the effort.

Professional bodies

Professional bodies usually arrange insurance for their members with insurance companies who understand their needs. They will certainly require evidence of insurance as part of the membership arrangements.

Useful websites

Australia

http://www.apra.gov.au/

Australian Prudential Regulation Authority (APRA)

Canada

Many websites are bilingual.

http://www.clhia.ca/index_en.htm

Canadian Life and Health Insurance Association

http://www.osfi-bsif.gc.ca/

Office of the superintendent of Financial Instructions of Canada
Governmental body implementing legislation in the insurance industry generally.

New Zealand

Governmental websites are bilingual.

http://www.acc.co.nz/

Accident Compensation Corporation
Their workplace cover provides injury cover for employees who suffer a work-related injury.

http://www.fpia.org.nz/

Financial Planners and Insurance Advisors Association

UK

http://www.fsa.gov.uk/

Financial Services Authority

USA

http://www.aicpcu.org/

American Institute for Chartered Property Casualty Underwriters and the Insurance Institute of America

http://www.cfp-board.org/

Certified Financial Planner

http://www.fpanet.org/

Financial Planning Association

http://www.naic.org/index.htm

National Association of Insurance Commissioners
These are insurance regulators and cover all the states. Database available on insurers.

Contracts 7

Chapter contents

Why contracts are necessary

Right from the start it is important to draft a comprehensive and well-thought-out contract, rather than find out you have an unforeseen problem later on when you have become embroiled in legal proceedings.

Some professional bodies have examples of sample contracts and this can be a useful starting point, but for peace of mind it is advisable to hire the services of a solicitor before signing or creating a contract.

If you are drafting a contract, it is important to produce a written list of your requirements. This will prevent you forgetting important issues when talking to a solicitor. A good solicitor who is experienced in commercial law will be able to convert your needs into a workable document, while adding any items necessary and explaining the contract to you.

A solicitor's time is expensive, so be sure of exactly what it is you want before you see one and read through the completed contract carefully before you discuss it with your solicitor.

It is important to take time to read the contract properly. Read it out loud, as this will prevent you missing relevant items and allow you to appreciate the document properly.

Contracts such as a licence for a practitioner to work within a room or premises are very straightforward and may not require this level of attention unless you are the person creating the contract.

Hiring employees

It is worth mentioning here that the wording of an advertisement for the purpose of hiring staff is very important. This is not only because of possible infringement of antidiscrimination legislation, but because a correct job description is very important. While consulting a solicitor on contracts, it is good idea to check that the advertisement you are going to place is suitable for your purposes.

Employee contracts

The moment an applicant accepts your offer of a job unconditionally is the moment the contract of employment starts.

The terms of the contract can be verbal, written, implied or a mixture of all three.

Even if you do not use a written contract, you are legally obliged to provide employees with a written statement of employment within 2 months of their starting work. This is not a contract, but provides evidence of the terms and conditions of employment between you and the employee if there is a dispute later on.

The written statement should include such items as:

- The names of the employer and the employee.
- The date when the employment (and the period of continuous employment) began.
- Remuneration and the intervals at which it is to be paid.
- Hours of work.
- Holiday entitlement.
- Entitlement to sick leave, including any entitlement to sick pay.
- Pensions and pension schemes.
- The entitlement of employer and employee to notice of termination.
- Job title or a brief job description.
- Where it is not permanent the period for which the employment is expected to continue, or if it is for a fixed term, the date when it is to end.
- Place of work.

The statement also has to:

- Cover any disciplinary rules which apply to the employee.
- Give a job description.
- Provide details of arbitration.

The Business Link website (see p. 70) has a page that allows you to construct a written statement specifically for your business.

As already stated, the terms of a contract of employment may be verbal, written, implied or a mixture of all three. They can be found in:

- The original job advertisements.
- A letter.
- Agreements.
- Staff rules.

Oral contracts are as binding as written ones, but if there is a dispute the terms of the contract may be difficult to prove.

A written contract leaves nothing to doubt and is similar in content to a written statement, but is signed by both parties and a copy retained by each.

If you want to change an existing contract, you will need to get your employee's written consent to the changes, or a breach of contract may take place and the employee could resign and claim constructive dismissal. The same principle applies to a written statement.

Associate contracts

This contract is specifically written for a self-employed person working from your premises and fulfils the criteria required by the tax office for someone to be self-employed. It is possible that your professional body has a copy of this type of contract for you to use as a template.

This type of contract needs the joint attention of a solicitor and an accountant, or a solicitor who is very conversant with tax law.

Rental contracts and licences

Property licence

You may find that taking out a substantial rental agreement may not suit you initially because you are looking for a more suitable premises, or the thought that you are entering a very binding financial contract for a long period of time is too daunting. In this case, taking out a licence with the landlord could be a suitable alternative. This may be for a suite of rooms or a single room.

A licence is far less binding than a rental contract and is less of a commitment than a rental agreement. It gives some security and guidelines for both the landlord and the person who is occupying the accommodation. Usually the termination period is 1 month's notice for either side. Do check, before you take on the licence, the reason why the landlord is prepared to terminate the agreement at such short notice. You do not want to establish a profitable clinic and settle in only to find that there are plans in a few months to change its usage entirely, leaving you with very little time to find other premises from which to work.

There is another element of instability with such a short-term agreement in that rent rises may occur far more rapidly than in a rental agreement.

Check to see what the fixed period is before the rent can be raised, as it may be as short as a month.

Many premises where a licence is involved may provide such services as receptionists or even secretarial services. Check to see what services are offered on the licence and see if these services are all-inclusive or require an extra payment. This may be a good way of having staff without needing to become involve in any financial or legal responsibility for them.

Do talk to the existing tenants to get an idea of how well the system works.

The licence should include:

- *Your liabilities.* How much per month the licence fee is and when it is to be paid. It is usual for services such as lighting, heating, etc. to be included in the terms of the licence. It will also include any extra services you are paying for, such as secretarial, receptionist, use of the telephone.
- *What you are allowed to do.* This may specify the therapy you are allowed to perform. Any additional therapies will require a change of licence. You may also be limited to what you can do with the room or premises you are in, e.g. you may not be able to change the structure of the building in anyway.

Rental lease

This is far more complex than a licence and requires a much longer-term commitment.

Before you decide to take on a particular property you will need information to work with:

- *Compare the premises you are likely to be renting with others,* not only for rent but also service charges and rates, etc. There may be hidden costs involved such as registration fees, or legal costs.
- *The premises must be legally owned by whomever you are renting from* or that person must have the legal means to rent the premises to you (see assigning on or subletting, below).
- *Are the premises unoccupied?* Can you be prevented from entering them by a current tenant?
- *Is there anything in the building* such as furniture and, if you do not want it, who will remove it?
- *Are the measurements of the premises accurate?* Rents are largely based on charges per square metre. If the measurement is smaller than listed on the rental documents then you may be entitled to renegotiate a more favourable price.
- *Are there any planning restrictions or permission required?* You must also check before you take up a lease that there are no planning restrictions or planning permission required for a clinic.

In the lease itself you will need to check the following:

- *What is the period of the lease?* Leases can last from 1 year to 20 years or more. Short leases can be obtained but generally landlords are not keen on these, since it is much easier and more financially secure to have a long-term tenant.
- *What are the restrictions on the property?* Are you limited as to the type of therapies you can perform or the amount of internal structural alterations?
- *How much of the repairs will you be required to perform?* Too many repairs will not make this a financially viable proposition. You need to avoid a fully repairing lease, as this will require you to make repairs to the fabric of the building, which could be very costly.
- *What service charges are involved?* If you are in a shared property there are very likely to be service charges. They are paid in advance with the rent to build up a fund for general maintenance, security, cleaning, etc. and for any emergency repairs that arise. This will add to the cost, but should mean someone else deals with maintenance without you personally incurring extra costs.
- *What are your basic rights?* Do you have unlimited access to the premises? Do you share any facilities, e.g. toilet? Can you put up signage? Do not forget that the landlords will also have certain rights, for instance if they need access to the premises if any work has to be done to it, but the amount of access should not create a nuisance.
- *Are you able to sublet?* You may want other practitioners in the premises to pay for some of the running costs, or simply want a multidisciplinary clinic.
- *Is there an option to assign?* You may want to leave the premises for whatever reason and find someone to take over. An option to assign allows you to pass the lease on to another business. Do check the legal position on your financial liability for this if the other business does not pay the rent for some reason.
- *Is there a break clause?* This is an option for either you or the landlord to terminate the lease early. If this is a possibility, you need to see how much notice to give. You also need to check if there are any particular conditions to exercising this option. The landlord may be entitled to refuse to accept the break if you breach any terms of the lease. If you do not have to give notice you may have to pay a certain number of months rent in lieu. It may be an idea to write into the lease the possibility of subletting or having an option to assign. This will mean that if you do not wish to use the premises, then you will still remain financially viable until your lease runs out.
- *When are the rent review dates?*
- *What will the review be based on?* Landlords generally use the following measures, although other methods are available:
    - *Open market rent.* This is the rent that the landlord could reasonably expect to obtain in the open market if he were letting the premises on a new tenancy on the same terms as the present tenancy.

  - *Changes in the Retail Price Index.* These are a measure of the changes in the prices at which retailers dispose of their goods to consumers and end-users. They can be found online in the Office for National Statistics website (see p. 70).
- *What happens if you do not agree?* It is very useful to make provision in a lease agreement for arbitration should any disputes between yourself and the landlord take place. Rent may be one of these issues. This can save you a great deal of expense going to court (see Arbitration, below).
- *Can you negotiate the future rent in advance if a rent review is due in the near future?*
- *Are you required to provide a personal guarantee?* Try to avoid a rental that involves this. If your business fails, then you will be liable for the rent and for any other payments due under the terms of the lease. This will be for the rest of the lease period.
- *Will you be required to pay a deposit?* When can you expect it to be repaid? Under what circumstances can the landlord keep some or all of it?
- *What will happen when the lease expires?* Providing you have elected to be covered by the Landlord and Tenant Act 1954, you will have a right to apply for renewal.

The Landlord and Tenant Act 1954 Part 2 was reformed in 2004 to give more protection to business tenants under the law. A booklet entitled 'Business tenancies: new procedures under the Landlord and Tenant Act 1954, Part 2' gives guidance on the new procedures for ending and renewing business tenancies.

Arbitration

This is a process that can be undertaken by a landlord and tenant to resolve a problem. It provides an alternative to going to court. By referring any dispute to a third and impartial party, who is usually an expert in the field, it saves both parties great expense.

The object according to the Arbitration Act 1996 is to:

- Obtain a fair resolution of disputes by an impartial tribunal without unnecessary delay or expenses.
- Allow both parties a certain freedom to agree on how the dispute is to be solved.

In an arbitration dispute both parties are jointly responsible for any costs that arise out of it.

Conclusion

The contents of this chapter are designed to be thought provoking and an introduction to some of the legal complexities of the contracts that you may undertake. They are a guideline and it is generally a good idea to seek the advice of a commercial solicitor to guide you through the process. A solicitor will not only be able to draw up a contract, but will be able to explain any problematical omissions or other difficult areas.

Unless you are very experienced in this area, it is better to let a solicitor draft a contract for you. This should not be exorbitantly expensive and may be money well spent later on if there is a dispute. It should be possible to get a quotation for this type of work before you engage a solicitor.

Useful websites

Australia

http://www.business.gov.au/Business+Entry+Point/

Australian Government

http://www.industrialrelations.nsw.gov.au/

Office of Industrial Relations New South Wales

http://www.lawcouncil.asn.au/about.html

The Law Council of Australia

http://www.ocba.sa.gov.au/tenancies/

Australian Government
Information on tenancies with links to different governmental areas of Australia.

Canada

Many websites are bilingual.

http://bsa.cbsc.org/gol/bsa/site.nsf/en/index.html

Canadian Government Business Start-up Assistant
Arranged by territories and provinces.

http://www.cba.org/CBA/Gate.asp

Canadian Bar Association

http://www.flsc.ca/

Federation of Law Societies of Canada
National coordinating body for all 14 law societies in Canada.

New Zealand

Governmental websites are bilingual.

http://www.biz.org.nz/public/Section.aspx?SectionID=46&FromSectionID=7

Business Information Zone
Site for information on employing staff.

http://www.nz-lawsoc.org.nz/

New Zealand Law Society

UK

http://www.businesslink.gov.uk

Business Link

http://www.lawsociety.org.uk

Law Society of England and Wales

http://www.lawscot.org.uk

Law Society of Scotland

http://www.lawsoc-ni.org/

Law Society of Northern Ireland

http://www.statistics.gov.uk/

Office for National Statistics

USA

http://www.dol.gov/

US Department of Labor
Information on various aspects of employment.

Reference

Office of the Deputy Prime Minister, London. 2004 Business tenancies: new procedures under the Landlord and Tenant Act 1954, Part 2. Available: http://www.odpm.gov.uk/pub/329/BusinesstenanciesnewproceduresundertheLandlordandTenantAct1954PDF430Kb_id1128329.pdf

Legislation

8

Chapter contents

Any therapists qualifying from a reputable college should have a reasonable awareness of the state of legislation associated with their respective professions and will be more than likely kept up to date with the ever-changing situation in this difficult legal area.

Each association issues guidelines to ensure the standard of behaviour they expect from their members. In the case of chiropractors and osteopaths there is a legal obligation to follow the rules laid down by their respective registers.

As well as legislation directly related to professional standards there is legislation affecting the workplace. The acquisition of employees will markedly affect the appreciation you will need to have of the various rules and regulations.

Unfortunately, because of the sheer volume of different legislature, it is easy to fall foul of it and you may only discover this to your cost when a mishap occurs. The various examples of legislation below should give you as a new business owner a feeling for areas that may require your attention.

General

Health and Safety at Work Act 1974

The key facts to note are the five responsibilities:

1. To make sure equipment does not damage health.
2. To make sure goods on the premises are safe; for example, no access to potentially poisonous herbs, unless the person concerned is qualified to handle them.
3. To inform, train and supervise staff.
4. To make sure the premises are safe and have the appropriate emergency exits.
5. To make sure the environment is safe and has necessary facilities.

If the place of work has over nine employees then an accident book is necessary; however, it may be a useful means of keeping an accurate record of an event even if you only have one employee.

Local Government (Miscellaneous Provisions) Act 1982

This act applies to acupuncturists, and chiropractors performing dry needling. Both are required to register themselves with the Local Authority.

Mostly, the respective authorities will have application forms available on the Internet with instructions for payment and delivery of the form. You will then receive a visit from a local government official who specializes in this type of licensing. The room in which you are performing your treatment will be inspected, and you will be required to answer a short questionnaire, which may consist of questions about how you are going to keep your couch clean and dispose of your sharps.

You will find the Local Authority is there to help you, not obstruct you, and you may find their comments helpful if you need to make adjustments to the room in order to obtain your certificate.

If they are satisfied with the arrangements, you are usually given permission to practice immediately and a licence will arrive shortly afterwards. This has to be displayed in a visible place.

The key points usually checked are cleanliness and disposal of needles into a sharps box.

Management of Health and Safety at Work Regulations 1999

A written statement of health and safety is required in a workplace with over five employees. Any establishment with fewer than five employees is exempt.

Something to note if you do expand your business is that if you own more than one clinic and the total number of employees is over five then you will be required to write a health and safety policy statement.

The policy is usually written in three parts:

1. *Statement of intent.* This shows what you will be required to do to manage health, safety and the environment effectively, so that you know what standard you have to achieve.
2. *Organization.* This states who is responsible for which aspect of health and safety.
3. *Arrangements.* This explains how you are going to perform your statement of intent.

Workplace (Health Safety and Welfare) Regulations 1992

These concern keeping equipment in good order and ensuring that the environment of the workplace is safe, clean and pleasant to work in. This can be something as simple as not letting the clinic get too hot or cold and ensuring that the general cleanliness is good.

In line with this legislation, practitioners must now have their equipment checked at least once a year by a company qualified to check the safety of both mechanical and electrical equipment, for example couches and ultrasound equipment.

Manual Handling Operations Regulations 1992

Although this is not a common consideration for a clinic, it may be possible from time to time that a disabled patient has to be assisted, or substantial deliveries arrive which require lifting.

Control of Substances Hazardous to Health (COSHH) Regulations 2002

Using chemicals or other hazardous substances at work can put people's health at risk. Although it is very unlikely that chiropractors opening their own premises would engage in setting up their own X-ray unit, this piece of legislation is worth noting for the future. Processor tank fluids are covered by this Act.

A certain amount of processor fluid will be washed into the drainage system by the processing unit, but large amounts should be disposed of responsibly. It is also important to take care of disposing of fixer. If any processor fluid is going down the drain, there has to be a silver filter on the drain inlets. Any responsible supplier of X-ray equipment and consumables will be able to advise you on how to comply with this legislation.

Acupuncturists or chiropractors who use disposable needles generate clinical waste and sharps that may be classified as hazardous because they are potentially infective. They are, however, exempt from needing to register with the Environment Agency annually if they produce less than 200 kg per annum of hazardous waste in total from the entire premises. If you work in a multidisciplinary clinic, it is unlikely that it will produce this amount of waste in a year, but you need to check this with the owner.

You will also be exempt if you work in a situation such as a doctor's surgery, educational establishment or from premises used by a charity.

It may be that the waste management company removing your waste may ask for evidence of your exemption, but this is unlikely as it will be obvious that you are not capable of producing over 200 kg per year of hazardous waste.

Ionising Radiation Regulations 1999

These lay out the requirements for correct use of ionizing radiation and minimizing risk.

If your X-ray machine is installed by a reputable company, it should be working closely with the radiation protection advisor you appoint to ensure you are maximizing the effectiveness of your equipment without compromising the patient.

It is worth being aware of this legislation even if you do not have X-ray equipment. If you are a chiropractor or osteopath you may need a colleague to produce a set of X-ray films for you.

Ionising Radiation (Medical Exposure) Regulations 2004

These are to ensure that there is justification for exposing a person to ionizing radiation.

Provision and Use of Work Equipment Regulations 1998

The relevance to practitioners is the requirement to ensure that equipment such as couches, lasers and ultrasound equipment is in good working order and not dangerous to other practitioners, staff or patients.

Equipment associated with taking and processing X-rays is covered under the Ionising Radiation Regulations 1999 and is serviced by a specialized engineer.

Other equipment should be serviced annually by engineers who understand the structural and electrical qualities of the treatment equipment.

Registration of Class 3 or Class 4 lasers

As yet the position is still being confirmed by the various professional bodies, which may be able to gain an exemption; otherwise individual members are required by law to register with the Healthcare Commission.

Personal Protective Equipment at Work Regulations 1992

Protective equipment may include an overall and goggles (if necessary) to protect someone changing processor fluid in an X-ray processor.

Health and Safety (Display Screen Equipment) Regulations 1992

This particular piece of legislation is more applicable to people working exclusively on a computer all day with very little break, a situation that would be unusual for a receptionist.

If you do think any of your employees are likely to be seated in front of a computer screen for some time then you may have to take measures to facilitate its safe use.

Electricity at Work Regulations 1989

These necessitate any electrical appliances (except X-ray equipment) being checked for safety once a year by a qualified electrician (see Ch. 5). The wiring of the buildings should be checked every 5 years.

A worksheet will indicate what appliances have passed the test and those that have not. All appliances passing the test are issued with a sticker which shows when the appliance was checked and when the next test is due.

Health and Safety (First Aid) Regulations 1981

Any staff injuries must be reported to the person in charge, and any serious ones to the Health and Safety Executive (HSE) or you are breaking the law. The accident is recorded in an accident book. A leaflet concerning this part of the Act is available from the HSE website (see p. 84). The leaflet details the factors that should be considered in a risk assessment. It contains more aspects than are required in a clinic but acts as a useful guideline.

The minimum first aid provision at any place of work should be:

- A correctly stocked first aid box.
- An appointed person to take charge of first aid arrangements.

The *appointed person* may not have had full first aider training, but will be able to take charge of someone who is injured or becomes ill, and will be the person to arrange for the ambulance to be called.

A *first aider* will have undergone a training course in administering first aid at work and will hold a current first aid at work certificate, from an organization that has been approved by the HSE. This certificate has to be renewed every 3 years.

Basically, as far as clinics are concerned, the examples of issues brought up in the leaflet that might be considered are as follows:

- *Make a brief assessment of any significant risks in the workplace.* An acupuncturist needs to assess how to store and dispose of needles safely, so that no one in the clinic either as a practitioner or visitor comes into contact with them. X-ray equipment emits radiation while in use. The use of kitchen equipment such as kettles may be an issue.
- *Are there any specific risks?* For example, a herbalist stocking herbs that can only be dispensed by a qualified practitioner should provide special secure storage to prevent unauthorized people gaining access to them. A chiropractor with X-ray equipment needs to note both the equipment and the processing fluid, since both may be though of as hazardous substances.
- *Are there parts of your establishment where different levels of risk can be identified?* The X-ray unit of a chiropractic clinic presents a higher level of risk than the reception area.
- *What is your record of accidents and cases of ill-health?* What type are they and where did they happen? This is fairly low risk in any clinic as there is no large machinery, but something such as a needle-stick accident has to be noted. One of your staff or colleagues may spill boiling water over herself, while making a hot drink.
- *How many employees are present on site?* In the case of a clinic there may be very few, but it may be a good idea to have someone familiar with basic first aid. This person may be yourself, although your receptionist could also be trained.
- *Are there inexperienced workers on site, or employees with disabilities or special health problems?* Do you have to make any special arrangements for them?
- *Do you have employees on the premises who work alone?* This may occur only when a practitioner goes out for lunch, in which case an attack is more likely than an accident.

- *Do any of your employees work at sites occupied by other employers?* This may probably be relevant if you are working in managed accommodation.
- *Do you have any work experience trainees?* Clinics do occasionally have requests from schools for their pupils to visit the clinic. You will be sent a risk assessment sheet.
- *Do members of the public visit your premises?* This is always going to be so if you are running a clinic.

Generally speaking clinics are likely to come into the low-risk category.

It is a good idea to have a suitable first aid kit and ensure that the people in your clinic know what to do if someone incurs an injury or becomes seriously ill. This could be done with a simple briefing and by ensuring that clearly typed instructions are put in each room of the clinic. The instruction may be just to ring the emergency services for an ambulance stating the details of location and the patient's condition.

First aid training with a view to certification can be done by St John Ambulance or the Red Cross. There are also companies that run recognized first aider courses, which can be held at your clinic, at a time of your choosing.

If you work within someone else's establishment, then it may be worth checking that they have the correct provision for first aid and make sure you know where the first aid kit is and who the first aider is.

Even if you work on your own, it is worth buying a proper first aid kit that can stored where it is easily to hand.

Reporting of Injuries, Diseases and Dangerous Occurrences Regulations 1995

These are usually more applicable to dangerous workplaces such as mines, but there is scope for the reporting of repetitive injury and probably maintaining an accident report book.

Fire Precautions (Workplace) Regulations 1997

As stated in Chapter 5, once you have applied for planning permission, it is likely you will receive a visit from the a representative of the local fire brigade.

You can also call in an approved supplier of fire-detection and fire-fighting equipment who will also tell you what you will need and be able to supply the correct equipment and signage. Not only will you need appropriate extinguishers, but also the correct exit signage to allow someone to see the way to the exit in poor visibility due to smoke.

If you do not follow this helpful advice and a fire does occur, not only may your insurance be null and void, but you may also find yourself in court if there has been a serious injury or loss of life. The financial consequences are bad enough, even if your conscience has not been affected.

Furniture and Furnishings (Fire) (Safety) Regulations 1988 (as amended)

Ensure that your office and clinic furniture complies with these regulations. All new furniture should do so. If you are buying second-hand, check these details with the place from which you are buying the furniture.

New furniture should carry two labels, one permanent, the other a swing ticket. The ticket gives basic notice of compliance with fire tests and carries the warning 'Carelessness causes fire'.

If in doubt check with your Trading Standards Office (website, p. 86).

Disability Discrimination Act (DDA) 1995

This Act also applies in Northern Ireland. It consists of three parts and aims to end the discrimination that disabled people have faced.

The Act gives disabled people rights in three main areas:

- Employment.
- Access to goods, facilities and services.
- Buying or renting land or property.

It is largely the first two areas, employment and access to goods, facilities and services, that may affect most therapists, although if you do have premises and do not consider the request of a disabled therapist to work you might be contravening the Act.

The premises you are in should now be designed to cater for the disabled, who should be able to have easy access your premises. Access includes toilets, car parking and information as well as access to the treatment rooms.

Some professional bodies produce Braille leaflets, but they are expensive. It will be worth purchasing one, however, and asking patients to return it once they have read it. If you are not able to obtain Braille information leaflets then record your clinic leaflet and treatment information so it can be listened to.

If you are wanting to rent you will have to locate your practice on the ground floor, or have lift access to the floor you are on and provide a wheelchair ramp if necessary. You may want to make it a condition of renting that correct access has be provided before you are prepared to rent.

There are no exemptions, no matter how small the practice. Lack of funds is also not an excuse for not complying with the Act, although it is possible that if you are able to offer a house call then this would be a way of dealing with the problem of inaccessibility.

There is an accessible version of the Disability Discrimination Act on the website of the UK government's policy division (see p. 87), which is a resource for advice, legal and policy information relating to disability in the UK.

Race Relations Act 1976

This defines discrimination on the grounds of race.

Sex Discrimination Act 1975

This Act defines discrimination on grounds of sex.

There is a great deal of legislation that may be applicable to the practitioner, but this should be covered by employment contracts and the right of everyone to have fair treatment from another person regardless of who they are.

Patients

Data Protection Act 1984

This act requires anyone who keeps computerized personal information on other people to register with the Data Protection Registrar.

At the moment, practitioners using an entirely paper record-keeping system are excluded, but it is worth considering what information you may have such as letters and mailing databases you may retain on your clinic computer.

Once you have applied, you will be sent a form that will allow the Registrar to categorize your usage of the information you have.

This Act also gives your patients the right of access to the information being held on them in order to check its accuracy. It is also one of the reasons that, providing patients have authorized it, you should be able obtain a copy of their X-ray films from hospitals and their X-rays or possibly blood test reports from their GP. Making copies of X-ray films will always incur a charge for materials. The GP or other practitioner also has a right to charge for the service of providing copies, but due to professional courtesy this does not normally occur.

If you are not sure whether or not you have to register, check the Information Commissioner's website (see p. 87). You will be able to register your clinic online or by post.

Consumer Protection Act 1987

A consumer can sue any person who puts his or her name to a product if a defective product causes death, injury or damage to property valued at more than £275.

The suppliers or producers of the goods are liable unless they can prove that they did not supply the goods. This is also the case in the instance of herbal products packaged by a manufacturer. If the practitioner has bought the herbs from an approved supplier in good faith and there has been a problem because the product was faulty, e.g. there have been adulterants present, then blame is passed on down the chain to the manufacturer.

Sale and Supply of Goods Act 1994

- *The product you sell must be of satisfactory quality.* Anything such as back supports, herbs or nutritional supplements must be adequate for the job they are intended to perform.
- *They must be fit to sell.* If the goods have a shelf life, as in the case of herbs and nutritional supplements, then they must not be out of date.
- *They must be fit for the purpose for which they are being sold.* For example, if qualified herbal practitioners are allowing a loose herb, or tincture prescription, to be dispensed to their patients, then they are not contravening this Act if the herbs are acknowledged as being appropriate for the condition.
- *They must correspond with the description.* This can be open to interpretation, as herbal remedies do not always work, and dispensed loose herbs or tinctures made up by the herbalist do not usually come within this remit.
- *Services must be rendered with reasonable skill and reasonable care.* These aspects are usually covered by codes of professional ethics.
- *Services must be supplied within a reasonable time.* This may include something such as sending out a receipt a patient has requested.

Do not forget that the terms of this Act also apply to you as a consumer.

Trade Descriptions Act 1968

You cannot make outrageous claims for the efficacy of your treatment, such as curing cancer.

Consumer Act 1987

This details product liability, should a person become ill or injured through the purchase of a product.

Herbs and supplements

Buying from reputable suppliers, can prevent you selling anything that is dubious or against the law.

Each herbal association issues a list of herbs that are prohibited or endangered, and the suppliers will be aware of this. They will have a member of staff who may be a herbalist, who is up to date on all new legislation and directives.

A reputable supplement supplier that deals only with professionals usually has a member of staff well versed in legislation and the way in which the supplements are put together and work.

Conclusion

Generally speaking, many of these regulations will be covered by common sense. For instance you would not want someone tripping up on a worn piece of carpet or using toilet facilities that are unsanitary. In other words, the sort of care required is the same is as you should take whenever inviting someone into your home.

In other people's premises it is a good idea not to take anything for granted. To ensure your safety and your patients' safety you may want to check on the following:

- *Is there easy access for patients who may be disabled?*
- *Is the place clean?*
- *Is the equipment checked once a year and well maintained?* This will include items such as ultrasound equipment, couches and other therapeutic equipment.
- *Has adequate electrical testing been performed?* This will be for items such as lamps, kettles, refrigerators and other domestic electrical equipment. Is the wiring of the building checked every 5 years?
- *Is a current health and safety poster displayed?*
- *Are the fire exits clearly marked?*
- *Are there an adequate number of fire extinguishers and are they marked properly?*
- *Is there adequate sharps disposal and are containers replaced regularly?*

Make sure that if your are working from home, you do not end up with your house being classed as business premises, as the rates are different and more expensive than domestic Council Tax.

It is unusual for a clinic to receive a visit from a health and safety inspector, as the situation is so low risk. Should one call, the Health and Safety Executive website (see below) has useful information on what to expect.

If you are not sure, it is a good idea to take legal advice to avoid a problematical situation occurring.

Useful websites

Australia

Consultation with professional body should provide correct information regarding registration, usage of needles and sharps disposal.

http://www.accc.gov.au/content/index.phtml/itemId/3669

Australian Competition and Consumer Commission
Business rights and obligations.

http://www.act.gov.au/CAP/accesspoint/jsp?action=menuHome

Australian Capital Territory: Government

http://www.australia.gov.au/

Australian Government

http://www.caba.nt.gov.au/

Northern Territory: Government
Justice and consumer affairs.

http://www.comcare.gov.au/publications/factsheets/fact-sheet-4.html

Australian Government
Guide to Commonwealth occupational health and safety regulation and codes of practice.

http://www.consumer.tas.gov.au/

Tasmania: Government Department of Justice
Deals with consumer affairs.

http://www.consumer.vic.gov.au/CA256EB5000644CE/HomePage?ReadForm&1=Home~&2=~&3=~

Victoria: Government
Deals with consumer affairs.

http://www.docep.wa.gov.au/

Government of Western Australia
Consumer and employment protection.

http://www.fairtrading.act.gov.au/Traders_Main.html

Australian Capital Territory
Fairtrading website with relevant legislation for commerce.

http://www.fairtrading.nsw.gov.au/corporate/relatedsites/australiangovernmentdepartments.html

New South Wales Office of Fair Trading

http://www.fairtrading.qld.gov.au/oft/oftweb.nsf

Queensland Office of Fair Trading

http://www.lawaccess.nsw.gov.au/

New South Wales: Government
Law access online. Legal information and advice services.

http://www.nohsc.gov.au/

Australian Government Department of Employment and Workplace Relations. Office of the Australian Safety and Compensation Council

http://www.nsw.gov.au/

New South Wales: Government

http://www.nt.gov.au/

Northern Territory: Government

http://www.ocba.sa.gov.au/

Government of South Australia Office of Consumer and Business Affairs

http://www.qld.gov.au/

Queensland: Government

http://www.business.act.gov.au/businesslicences

Australian Capital Territory
Business licence information service.

http://www.sa.gov.au/site/page.cfm

South Australian Central Government

http://www.tas.gov.au/

Tasmanian Government

http://www.treasury.gov.au/content/consumer_affairs.asp?ContentID=270&titl=Consumer%20Policy

Australian Government
Website for consumer affairs.

http://www.vic.gov.au/

Victoria: Government

http://www.wa.gov.au/

Western Australia: Government

Canada

Many websites are bilingual.

http://www.bbb.org/

Better Business Bureau

http://bsa.cbsc.org/gol/bsa/site.nsf/en/index.html

Canadian government's start-up assistant
This covers all the territories. Extensive amount of information on legislation.

http://www.ccohs.ca/

Canadian Centre for Occupational Health and Safety
Resource website.

http://www.hrsdc.gc.ca/en/gateways/nav/top_nav/program/labour.shtml

Canadian Government
Labour program website. Contains useful information on various aspects of employment including legislation.

http://strategis.ic.gc.ca/epic/internet/inoca-bc.nsf/en/Home

Office of Consumer Affairs of Industry Canada

New Zealand

Governmental websites are bilingual.

http://www.acc.co.nz/

Accident Compensation Corporation
Their workplace cover provides injury cover for employees who suffer a work-related injury.

http://www.biz.org.nz/public/section.aspx?sectionid=36

Business Information Zone
Selected regulations for business.

http://www.biz.org.nz/public/section.aspx?sectionid=47&fromsectionid=29

Business Information Zone
Health and safety issues.

http://www.consumeraffairs.govt.nz/

Ministry of Consumer Affairs
Consumer advice and legislative information.

http://www.nz-lawsoc.org.nz/

New Zealand Law Society

UK

http://www.healthcarecommission.org.uk/Homepage/fs/en

Healthcare Commission

http://www.hse.gov.uk/

Health and Safety Executive

http://www.hse.gov.uk/pubns/hsc14.htm

Health and Safety Executive
Information on what to expect from a visit from a health and safety inspector.

http://www.opsi.gov.uk/

Office of Public Sector Information

Management of Health and Safety at Work Regulations 1999
http://www.opsi.gov.uk/si/si1999/19993242.htm

http://www.businesslink.gov.uk

Business Link
Information on health and safety

http://www.hse.gov.uk/lau/lacs/38-3.htm

Health and Safety Executive
Useful health and safety information in simplified form.

http://www.hse.gov.uk/pubns/indg259.pdf

Health and Safety Executive
Health and safety leaflet for small businesses.

Workplace (Health, Safety and Welfare) Regulations 1992
http://www.hse.gov.uk/lau/lacs/91-6.htm

Manual Handling Operations Regulations 1992
http://www.opsi.gov.uk/si/si1992/Uksi_19922793_en_1.htm

http://www.opsi.gov.uk/si/si1992/Uksi_19922793_en_4.htm

http://www.hse.gov.uk/lau/lacs/56-1.htm

Control of Substances Hazardous to Health (COSHH) Regulations 2002
http://www.hse.gov.uk/pubns/indg136.pdf

http://www.opsi.gov.uk/si/si2002/20022677.htm

http://www.coshh-essentials.org.uk/

Health & Safety Executive

http://www.environment-agency.gov.uk/subjects/waste/1019330/

Environment Agency

Ionising Radiation Regulations 1999
http://www.opsi.gov.uk/si/si1999/19993232.htm#13

Ionising Radiation (Medical Exposure) Regulations 2004
http://www.opsi.gov.uk/si/si2004/20041769.htm

Provision and Use of Work Equipment Regulations 1998
http://www.opsi.gov.uk/si/si1998/19982306.htm

Personal Protective Equipment at Work Regulations 1992
http://www.opsi.gov.uk/si/si1992/Uksi_19922966_en_1.htm

Health and Safety (Display Screen Equipment) Regulations 1992
http://www.opsi.gov.uk/si/si1992/Uksi_19922792_en_1.htm

Electricity at Work Regulations 1989
http://www.opsi.gov.uk/si/si1989/Uksi_19890635_en_1.htm

Health and Safety (First Aid) Regulations 1981
http://www.hse.gov.uk/pubns/indg214.pdf

http://www.redcrossfirstaidtraining.co.uk
British Red Cross

http://www.sja.org.uk/training/courses/workplace/
St John Ambulance

Reporting of Injuries, Diseases and Dangerous Occurrences Regulations 1995
http://www.opsi.gov.uk/si/si1995/Uksi_19953163_en_1.htm

Fire Precautions (Workplace) Regulations 1997
http://www.fire.org.uk/si/amd1840.htm

http://www.fireservice.co.uk/
Fire Service

http://www.bfsa.org.uk/
British Fire Services Association

http://www.nsi.org.uk/
National Security Inspectorate

Furniture and Furnishings (Fire) (Safety) Regulations 1988
http://www.opsi.gov.uk/si/si1989/Uksi_19892358_en_1.htm

http://www.tradingstandards.gov.uk/
Trading Standards

Disability Discrimination Act (DDA) 1995
http://www.opsi.gov.uk/acts/acts1995/1995050.htm

http://www.direct.gov.uk/DisabledPeople/fs/en

http://www.drc-gb.org/index.asp
Disability Rights Commission
Downloads of a Code of Practice: rights of access – goods, facilities, services and premises.

http://www.rnib.org.uk
Royal National Institute for the Blind

http://www.abilitynet.org.uk
Ability Net

Race Relations Act 1976
http://www.opsi.gov.uk/si/si2003/20031626.htm

Sex Discrimination Act 1975
http://www.opsi.gov.uk/

http://www.businesslink.gov.uk
Business Link

http://www.eoc.org.uk/
Equal Opportunities Commission

http://www.adviceguide.org.uk/index.htm
Citizens' Advice Bureau

Data Protection Act 1984
http://www.opsi.gov.uk/acts/acts1998/19980029.htm#aofs

http://www.informationcommissioner.gov.uk/eventual.aspx?id=34
Information Commissioner

Consumer Protection Act 1987
http://www.consumerdirect.gov.uk/general/unsafe/fs_d01.shtml

Sale and Supply of Goods Act 1994
http://www.opsi.gov.uk/acts/acts1994/Ukpga_19940035_en_1.htm

Trade Descriptions Act 1968
http://www.dti.gov.uk/files/file8156.pdf

Consumer Act 1987
http://www.dti.gov.uk/consumers/fact-sheets/page22855.html

Herbs and supplements
http://www.food.gov.uk/foodindustry/supplements

Food Standards Agency
Information on the European directive on food supplements.

http://www.bcma.co.uk/proposed_directive_on_traditiona.htm

British Complementary Medicine Association
Traditional herbal medicinal products directive.

http://www.herbsociety.co.uk/legislation.htm

Herb Society
Explanation of EU Medicines directive.

USA

Consultation with professional body should provide correct information regarding registration, usage of needles and sharps disposal.

http://www.dol.gov/

US Department of Labor
Information on various issues of rights regarding employment.

http://www.firstgov.gov/

United States Government

http://www.ftc.gov/

Federal Trade commission
Consumer rights website run by the government.

http://www.osha.gov/

US Department of Labor
Occupational safety and health administration.

Part 2

Marketing

Marketing introduction

9

Chapter contents

There is such a large amount of information published on marketing that it becomes overwhelming and much more complicated than a complementary practitioner setting up for the first time would need. Marketing is very important at any level of business, and the basic principles are the same for a small complementary practice as they are for a multinational company.

Marketing covers three main areas, all of which have equal importance and must be conducted properly if you are to understand the type of patient you are aiming to draw in, how to go about it and how to sustain a suitable patient load.

Marketing consists of:

- *Market research.* The research you do to understand who your patients are and where they are coming from.
- *Advertising.* The means to excite a potential patient's interest.
- *Public relations.* The interaction you and your clinic have with the patients in order to draw them into your treatment room and sustain a healthy patient load.

Even in a small business it is very necessary to grasp at least the basic skills of marketing. Having marketing skills allows you to understand where your business sits in the scheme of things and what you have to do to bring patients to you. Done properly, it should provide you with an objective viewpoint from which it will then be possible for you to make decisions enabling you to establish your business and move it forward. The information will also allow you to continue to make a good living even if there is an increase in competition.

Marketing enables you to match your service with the patients' needs. You must identify your customers and target them, because without them you have no business. Ultimately, successful treatments are only achieved because you have met the patient's needs.

Funding for the proposed venture will depend on how carefully you have researched your chosen patient population. Methodical marketing is very necessary to impress your potential lender, as the thoroughness of your research and careful analysis of the information you have gathered will show you have a sensible rationale.

Your lender will need to see a lucid argument for the direction in which you are going to take your business, and that you have considered what to do when times become financially challenging.

Your efforts in marketing are not just window dressing for your lender but, along with your financial considerations, will provide you with a yardstick by which you can measure the growth and degree of success of your business. They give you an appreciation of the world outside your clinic, and if the number of patients you are treating is not meeting your expectations, you will understand why and adjust your method of operation or expectations and finances accordingly.

If your business has exceeded all expectations, good marketing skills will prevent you from becoming complacent and allow you to analyse whether this is a trend that is likely to continue or whether you can expect fluctuations. Fine tuning your approach to drawing in patients will help in the expansion of your clinic.

For these reasons market research and analysis should be a regular exercise.

A thorough approach to marketing is essential for a new practitioner since it is possible that a deep immersion into studies over a long period of time could make you blinkered and unable to see yourself and your chosen therapy as the outside world does. The general public may have an entirely different perception of you and what you have to offer, and marketing allows you to consider your profession from an outsider's viewpoint. You will then be able to manage your public image properly, which is very important in building and maintaining a practice.

Marketing is usually done after you have developed your *business vision* (what you intend to do) and a good idea of what you will physically need to do it, for example premises, equipment, etc.

Once you have completed your marketing analysis from the information you have gathered, you will then be able to get a better idea if your vision needs to be adjusted in some way to make your clinic financially viable. This is no different from assessing a treatment plan and pursuing a different approach. Being a successful therapist relies a great deal on flexibility of mind. It is good to be single minded, but you must always have an appreciation that what you want may not be, certainly initially, practical.

The information you glean from your marketing exercise may also surprise you, and lead you off in an unexpected and equally rewarding direction to the one you originally intended, or give you useful leads which will bring about interesting developments you may not have considered.

Sources for market research

Market research does not need to be conducted at a high level by using a marketing firm or by you stopping people in the street with a questionnaire.

Very often you may find that students at the relevant colleges may have performed something akin to market research in a thesis, perhaps finding out public awareness of your particular therapy and how they perceive it. Your professional body may have also put money into such a survey or have used professionals who look for such research and may be able to direct you towards it.

There are also the occasional polls conducted by various newspapers and magazines, which might give you an idea of public perception of and attitudes towards your profession. Newspapers and magazines are also good sources of information. There is an ongoing process of articles being written on complementary medicine and this largely tends to reflect the public perception of complementary therapy. Do not be put of by articles that might not be favourable, since they will make you aware of negative perceptions you may face with the general public.

Marketing is an ongoing process, and one that you should, to a certain extent, be engaged in all the time. Visits to local shops may provide a wealth of information from looking at advertisements placed in windows to talking to the shopkeeper. It is also possible to keep in touch with the local scene through local newspapers, many of which are available (with a time delay of a day or so) on the Internet.

Once you have been trading for a while you can construct a questionnaire on patient satisfaction, which patients can fill in while waiting for you.

Market research will provide a road map, which allows you to see more clearly where you want to go with your business and the most efficient way to get there. Many businesses lose money because they do not understand their market and are directing the wrong product at the wrong people or are in a market that cannot support purchase of the product. In other words, you may be in an area of older people who do not want treatment for sports injuries or your prices may be too high. You will not know this unless you do your marketing.

Part of the marketing function will be to build your business image. There are ways of projecting your image without spending a fortune. It may well be that your potential patients may not want to walk into a dark and dreary clinic, but with a little more lighting and a new coat of an appropriate shade of paint on the walls, the place can be transformed and start to bring in the type of patient you have been wanting to treat, purely because they feel more comfortable because of the changes.

Summary

- Marketing consists of three elements:
  - Market research

- Advertising
- Public relations.

- Marketing matches the needs of the patient to the practitioner.
- The customer will always be at the centre of your business.
- Marketing is the vital link between you the practitioner and your patients.
- Create in yourself a sense of awareness of what is going on in the world around you and do not become complacent.

Market research 10

Chapter contents

Market research enables you to see if your business aim can be realistically achieved, since it is no good establishing a practice in a location that is not able to support you financially.

Once you are established, ongoing market research will be invaluable in keeping your business on an even keel by allowing you to assess whether your practice is matching your patients' needs and also whether expansion is appropriate.

It may be as simple as asking how the patient has found out about you, which can be done while filling out the personal details of a case history form. This information will allow you to build up a picture of which particular type of advertising seems to be the most effective way of alerting potential patients to your practice. It will also highlight the most inefficient methods, and prevent you spending unnecessarily on expensive advertising that is having no effect.

Patient feedback is important and may be worth pursuing after a few visits in the form of a questionnaire, which can be filled in while the patient is waiting to see you. This type of feedback is an invaluable way of letting you know if the clinic's services are meeting expectations.

Market research also enables you build up a comprehensive picture of your competitors and what space they occupy in the marketplace.

Mission statement

Market research is not a random collection of data, but a methodical line of enquiry that can only be performed by asking specific questions. Creating a mission statement is therefore not just a PR tool, but concisely defines the nature and standard of the service you provide.

Knowing how you wish to fit into the community as a practitioner will make your efforts in market research easier and much more efficient. The service you provide is after all a product and you will need to have a clear idea exactly what the product is you are marketing.

A mission statement succinctly describes the essence of your business. It should contain the function of your business and to whom the service is targeted.

Sorting out a mission statement is not only valuable for your business plan, but also your PR. Many people when asked what they do find themselves unable to easily express the nature of their job succinctly. A clear well-articulated statement shows you have carefully considered all the aspects of the service you have to offer and have a thorough understanding of what is involved. This will lend a great sense of professionalism to what you are able to offer and is an example of good PR.

Creating a mission statement is not easy, however, and requires some thought. Take some time aside, in a place where you are able to consider all the factors involved with your clinic, without interruption.

How do I go about creating a mission statement?

There are several questions you can ask yourself to help you through the process:

- *What is your chosen vocation?* This is the therapy you have trained in.
- *Who are you going to deliver the service to?* Your vision for your clinic and your market research should have decided this for you. Will it be a specialist area, for example the older population, or the more general population?
- *What is going to make patients come to you instead of your competitors?*
- *How do you want people to think of your clinic if it is brought up in conversation?* Obviously you want it to be seen in a positive light, but what are they going to say other than you are good? You may want them to say that your knowledge is extensive or you express great interest in their welfare.
- *What benefits do patients receive if they come to see you?* This is more than just wanting to 'cure' them. If you have patients who can never fully recover, you may seek to improve their quality of life. You may want to

give other patients management techniques that will keep them healthy for the rest of their life.

Once you have produced a mission statement give it to a relative or friend and get their feedback on it.

Define your area of research

There is an overwhelming amount of potential information out there. Some will be very relevant to you and the rest will be a complete waste of time and resources to pursue, even with help. So how do you narrow down your field of search?

Firstly consider the three main factors:

- You
- The patients
- Your competition, the other practitioners out there who are likely to be trying to attract the same type of patient as you are.

Your mission statement is also very helpful as it effectively identifies your target market. Knowing this allows you to pose questions that will provide you with relevant information and avoid wasting a great deal of your precious time.

You should then gather information, which identifies the following:

- *What is the size of the market in your chosen area?* If, for example, you have chosen to treat the elderly, how many live within accessible distance of the clinic?
- *Are their needs currently being met?* Are there any other therapists in the area and are they providing the type of treatment that you have already envisaged in your mission statement?
- *To what extent do you feel you will be able to gain your market share of patients?* What are you going to provide compared to your competitors that might make you more attractive?
- *What is your pricing structure going to be?* You will need to know what everyone else is charging.
- *How are you going to reach your target audience?* Look at what is available to you in magazines, newspapers, and professional leaflets.
- *What are the trends and potential changes which may impact on your market?* Garner information on legislation or government initiatives that may have an impact on your profession.
- *Where are the resources for finding out information?* How will you get this information?

Each question will more than likely have a subheading.

Where are you going to get your information?

Public resources

As already mentioned, there are considerable resources available from your local library and even online access if you do not have a computer. The Internet, however, is now one of the most popular ways of initially gathering information.

To get a feel for the area you wish to set up in, it is worth accessing a website such as the one run by the Office for National Statistics (see p. 108). This site covers a range of statistics associated with the UK and will enable to you get an idea of the type of people who live in the area you have chosen. You will be able to see information such as the percentage in each age range, level of employment, how many people occupy a dwelling, what type of accommodation is available and its cost. This is a good rough and ready way of assessing the economy of an area, before visiting the location. Every country has a National Statistics or National Census website.

Information available on the ground

General information

It is impossible to perform all your market research from the comfort of your own home, so if it is not well known to you, you will need to go out into the area you intend to work and get a feel for the place first hand. Even if you are local to the area, you may not appreciate how the atmosphere changes at different parts of the day.

The type of property will give you an idea of the income bracket of that area. Find a few that are for sale and check on their prices compared to the rest of the area. This is also possible to do on the Internet, but viewing the properties yourself will allow you to see exactly what the property looks like and where it sits in its environment.

Walk around to see how many people are out during the day. It may well be that you are going to establish your practice in an affluent area, but the place is like a ghost town during the day since everyone is away at work, so the only way you can make a living is by working at night and the weekend.

A certain economic group is likely to predominate in your chosen area. Find out what it is. Is it young professionals, families or retired people? Each group has different needs that you need to appreciate. This again can be done by general observation on the ground or from looking at the Office for National Statistics website.

If the area is non-residential, make a note of what businesses are around.

If it is a shopping centre:

- *How busy is it?* A busy shopping centre means that there is a large population of people available during the day for treatment.

- *What types of shops are there?* Are the goods being sold of the type that will bring people into the area from further away than the immediate neighbourhood? Will the goods on sale encourage them to take their time in the area?
- *What is the quality of goods for sale?* High quality, expensive merchandise, particularly for home decoration or in the area of speciality foods, suggest the residents in the neighbouring areas have the financial means to support this type of commerce.
- *What types of cafés or restaurants serve the area?* Again, a well-furnished café or restaurant and the type of food it is serving will indicate the economic level of the surrounding area.
- *What is the state of repair of the shops and their décor?* These details along with the types of goods available give a clear indication of the level of economy the area can sustain.
- *How long have the businesses been there?* If the shops look cosmetically wonderful, but have only been there a very short time, this can indicate two things. There is a rapid turnover in shops as the area cannot sustain them or this is an up-and-coming area with great potential.

In an area with offices:

- *Are they managed units or large single-occupation offices?* Managed units are usually found in economically depressed areas. Large single-occupation offices may well have the financial means to afford complementary treatment under contract.
- *What state of repair and decoration are the offices in?* As with the shops, this will indicate the economic level of the area.

It is worth bearing in mind that many large businesses have healthcare schemes and it is not unheard of for large businesses to buy in the services of a complementary therapist to either treat on site or at the clinic location.

Accessibility

You will be running a business that is only capable of making money if people physically visit it. So it is important to have an appreciation of how patients are going to get to your clinic.

How easy is it to get to your clinic?

- *Do the buses run frequently and are there stops nearby?*
- *How many changes is a patient going to have to make to get to you from various locations?*
- *Is it going to be too much trouble for the patients to get to you?*
- *How easy is it to park?* If you only have street parking available, do go back at different times of the day to make sure it is plentiful. Check also that the streets do not require a special parking permit. Occasionally local councils will change their policies on parking; is that likely to

happen near where you are? A street that is turned into an urban freeway at certain times of the day or suddenly acquires double yellow lines down its length will mean that patients may not be able to park outside your clinic and will be forced to park some way off before walking to you.

Local information

Being shy does not make a successful businessperson. If you do not ask questions you will never be able to get the information you want to know.

You have already acquired some local information from observation. Now it is necessary to start asking questions. It is not necessary to stop people in the street to do this, but while you are out shopping in the area you have chosen as the location of your practice, casual conversation can be very helpful in assessing the local market for your skills.

You may find out:

- If they have heard of your therapy.
- How much they understand about it.
- About your potential competitors.
- The general economy of the area.

Chatting to people you meet when the opportunity arises is also a very useful public relations exercise, and communication will, after all, be one of the most important factors for your success as a practitioner.

Your competitors

Information to be gained inside. It is worth going to see the premises of your potential competitors. Although many may not see your visit as a positive move on your part, there will be others who feel that announcing yourself is good manners, and as a result feel less hostile towards your opening up nearby. Meeting them face to face will give you a much better idea of:

- Who they are.
- How long they have been established.
- The type of service they see themselves providing.
- Their pricing structure.

Not only might you gain ideas and more precise information, but it enables you to see a range of premises from the viewpoint of a visitor and be able to assess how you react to them in that context. As with other businesses, the state of repair and décor will say a great deal about the proprietor of the clinic.

Information from external observation. Signage may tell you how long they have been established and about the therapies they have to offer.

If they have a car park is it constantly full? A general rule of thumb is that a clinic that has been in operation a long time and is successful should have a well-patronized car park and clinic.

If does not then there are two possibilities:

- They may not be matching the service they offer to patient needs.
- There may not be a market for that particular therapy in that area.

How wide a net should you cast?

When starting up a new clinic it is better to limit market research to your locality. There is no point conducting it on a nationwide basis, since patients are unlikely to visit you from a great distance.

Although you are concerned with your immediate surroundings, it is a good idea to get a grasp of economic trends nationally. The Office for National Statistics will enable to you get an idea of such factors as retail sales and employment, which affect the amount of money people have available to spend.

Additional research

As far as the complementary field is concerned the websites of the professional organizations, and the printed *Yellow Pages* and website, are probably the best places to start.

The websites of the various professional associations will give you names and locations and probably, in the same way as the Yell.com website, links to individual clinics where even more information may be available, such as the type of conditions they treat and the other therapies they have available, or even if they are part of a group of clinics. The quality of the advertisement and website alone may tell you a great deal about the budgets available to those clinics and the image they wish to project to the general public.

With any printed advertising look for:

- *The size of the advertisement and its quality.* A large clinic may support a larger advertisement, but this does not necessarily follow. The advertisements will give you an idea of what budget you will need to compete with the other clinics.
- *Where they are.* This will enable you, with the use of a town plan or map, to see how close other practitioners are likely to be to where you are contemplating setting up.
- *What professional body they belong to.* Is it the same as yours? If it is not, then what is the difference?
- *What they have to offer.* This may range from easy parking to evening clinics and free initial consultations. Some therapists may be qualified in more than one discipline.

Additional forms of advertising

Look at other advertisements that the other practitioners are taking out. These may be in local newspapers, parish magazines, local information publications, libraries or health food shops.

Generally speaking, therapists who are busy have very little advertising. The more consistently they advertise, the less likely they are to be busy, or they may be trying to expand their clinic.

Many practitioners produce their own leaflets. These may be found in local shops or cafés and restaurants, particularly if these outlets are specialist such as vegetarian or vegan. Leaflets can vary in quality, but as well as providing information, they will give you ideas for any leaflets you might produce in the future. They are also likely to give some pricing structure, which will be useful when you come to decide what prices you are going to charge.

Trade fairs

These can vary greatly in quality. It may be worth visiting one if it is run locally, just to see what is there and pick up more detailed information. It will certainly enable you to speak to practitioners face to face and get to know a little more about them on a personal level.

Market overview

This is a checklist of questions that will enable you to compile a picture of the market that you will be attempting to capture. It is not a definitive list, but a way of creating a logical method of accumulating information.

Size of market

- *What is the total market?* You need a rough idea of the population of your town/city or local area.
- *Who is likely to make up the majority of your patient base?* Are these likely to be the elderly, those with chronic diseases or a complete range of patients?
- *What distance are people likely to travel to see you?* As a new practitioner, accept that this is not likely to be very far. In a city it may be as little as a couple of miles owing to the problems of traffic; in the country the catchment area may extend to 10 miles or more.
- *What frequency of repeat visits are you likely to expect?* You will have an idea clinically of what is required to achieve an improvement and the amount of treatment to maintain this. Further research will enable you to ascertain what is actually viable.
- *Is the market growing or shrinking?* Is the economy affecting spending, or a sudden flood of practitioners into the area likely to make things difficult? Are you the only therapist of your kind in your locality, making it wide open for your therapy?

- *Is there likely to be a seasonal influence?* Is business likely to go down during holiday time, or increase with gardening injuries or the onset of the hay fever season?
- *Does your potential patient base understand the benefits of your therapy?* If they have increased awareness then it will be easier for you to access your market. Lack of awareness will leave the market wide open but will also mean that you will have to spend time educating your potential patients in order to bring them in.
- *Is your therapy prone to fads?* Some therapies are fortunate to be well established, others may increase or decrease in popularity according to the type of publicity they receive.
- *Are any factors likely to alter the market?* Many complementary therapies are seen as luxury items and are the first to go when the economy takes a downturn. In many case this is just a matter of re-educating the patients' perception of the benefit they can receive from occasional but continuing treatment.

  This information also creates a customer profile.

The competition

Analysis of your competitors will give you an idea of the market that is likely to be available to you.

- *Who are your main competitors and how big a part of the market are they capturing?* This will be an intelligent guess based on size of premises and the reconnaissance you have undertaken.
- *What range of therapies are they offering?* Can they do anything for patients that you cannot?
- *If they are busy, why is that?* Again, this may be derived from your knowledge of them within the profession and your reconnaissance.
- *What are their strengths and weaknesses?*
- *Where might you be able to surpass the competition?* You may have expertise in an area they do not, e.g. someone who originally trained as a midwife will have a wealth of information about dealing with mothers and babies that other people do not.
- *What are the trends?* Have any recent newspaper articles indicated interest in your particular therapy? Do not forget that local newspapers usually archive their material, which is available on the Internet. Local radio and TV all have websites with archived material.

You

- *How do you compare with the rest of the market?* Has your training been so in-depth that you will be ahead of the field when you start to treat? Is your inexperience likely to affect your street credibility?
- *Where are you likely to make the most profit and where do you see your growth.* If you have more than one therapy available, is one going to

make more money for you while the other works alongside it? How are you going to utilize your therapy to build your practice, e.g. are you going to concentrate on a particular condition?

- *Do you need to qualify in other areas to enhance your existing service?* You may need to undertake more training in another therapy that complements your primary one in order to level the competition.
- *Do you have a good location to work from?* Are you easily accessible? Is there parking? Do the premises look good?
- *How are you going to promote yourself?* You should now have a comparison with your competitors to see how your advertising can be more or just as effective.
- *What is the cost of marketing?* This will be largely advertising in print and on the Internet. It also includes cost of advertising at trade fairs, including travel and time away from the clinic.
- *Have you revised any original thoughts that you had on the way you see your business being presented?*

Your service

- *Who will use your service?*
- *How often are they likely to visit per week and how many visits do you envisage?* This will start to help you piece together patient numbers over a period of time.
- *Are you going to offer other therapies alongside the one you are already intending to use as your primary therapy?* This is where you may decide on a different pricing structure or whether the other therapy is appropriate at this stage.
- *What is the customers' perception of your therapy and how do you wish them to perceive your therapy?* Although not definitive research, your conversation with local people and investigation of the local media should have provided more information. You may only be able to change perception over a period of time, but if that is what you want to do then you must have a plan of action that is based on the research you have done and continue to perform.
- *Do you have a logo that will become associated with your clinic?* Many people react positively to a well-thought-out visual image. It may be worth paying for a graphic designer to create a logo that will be synonymous with you and give you a more professional image.
- *Is the price right?* Have you investigated the local pricing structure to see what the market will stand, but at the same time not under-price yourself?
- *Does your service have a life cycle?* In terms of marketing a product, which your service effectively is, are you dealing with a therapy that has previous displayed a fluctuation in popularity?
- *Do you need to train further?* This may be only something that can be answered as time goes on, but there is nothing worse than a practitioner who has become complacent and fixed in a set routine.

The patient

- *Who makes the decision regarding the need for treatment?* If you are dealing with families then it may well be the mother who makes this decision. If you are dealing with young professionals then you will have to appeal directly to them.
- *How can you reach them?* How are you going to make them aware of your presence? By talks, advertising, contacting the firm they work for?
- *What type of patient are you going to be treating?* Are they children, young executives, housewives, or older members of the population?
- *What are they likely to want from you in the way of treatment?* What sort of treatment are they expecting you to give them? Do they perceive it as a period of time or just a result? Do they think it is going to take a long time or produce an instantaneous result?

Conclusion

Marketing information is vital to your future – make sure that you are thorough. By giving yourself clear tasks and headings, the information you gain in your investigations should be easily accessible and understandable and allow you to move to the next phase of analysis.

Market research becomes much easier once you have been established, as you will be able to ask a wide range of patients directly about the services you offer.

The Chartered Institute of Marketing website (see below) has a few articles and useful definitions associated with marketing.

Useful websites

Australia

http://www.abs.gov.au/

Australian Bureau of Statistics

http://www.ami.org.au/

Australian Institute of Marketing
This website has a library of interesting marketing articles.

Canada

Many websites are bilingual.

http://www.cinstmarketing.ca/

Canadian Institute of Marketing
Resource page with magazine containing useful articles on marketing in PDF format.

http://www12.statcan.ca/english/census01/home/index.cfm

Census of Canada

New Zealand

Governmental websites are bilingual.

http://www.marketing.org.nz/

Marketing Association of New Zealand

http://www.salesmarketing.org.nz/

Sales and Marketing Institute of New Zealand
Various articles on marketing.

http://www.stats.govt.nz/default.htm

Statistics New Zealand

UK

http://www.cim.co.uk/cim/index.cfm

Chartered Institute of Marketing

http://www.statistics.gov.uk

Office for National Statistics

USA

http://www.census.gov/

United States Census Bureau

Analysing marketing information and preparing it for use

11

Chapter contents

Once you have completed your research and looked at every aspect of your business you will need to pull all this information together and analyse it. Your analysis will enable you to see if you are going to target the right sort of patient for your therapy and that you are establishing yourself in the right location. You will also be able to create a credible marketing plan, with a view to advertising and PR.

Analysing information is something you have done all your life. You have used it to buy a house or car and in deciding which therapy to train in. Now your analysis will require a more formal and focused approach.

Strengths, weaknesses, opportunities, threats (SWOT) analysis

A SWOT analysis is in a way an extension of thinking in terms of pros and cons. This type of analysis looks at your strengths and weaknesses compared to those of your competitors and considers the opportunities and threats that your competitors and the world outside your clinic present. By considering your business in this way you are identifying its positive points and acknowledging its flaws.

It is best to use short bullet points at this stage and not elaborate further, since you are creating a checklist to act on.

Strengths

These describe the positive qualities that are within your control and add value to your business or give you some edge over the competition. They will give some perspective of advantages you are likely to have over your competitors.

Try to examine what will make your clinic stand out to its advantage and encourage patients to visit you, as well as the resources you have available to help you run your clinic. This could be in terms of:

- Your abilities.
- The location of your clinic.
- The quality of your staff.
- Your education.
- The membership of your professional body giving you credibility.
- Contacts.
- Equipment you might already have.
- Savings you have available to use on the business.

Do not forget that your strengths may not come purely from you. It may well be that a relative or friend has expertise in a certain area, for example finance, or may have no more than an outgoing personality and the ability to engage people in conversation while performing some useful PR for your clinic.

Weaknesses

These are the negative factors within your control, which will reduce your ability to gain and maintain a competitive edge. Identifying these aspects will enable you to address these problems.

Weaknesses might be:

- Your lack of experience.
- Limited resources.
- Poor location.
- Not having staff to help you with administration.

What can you do to improve any deficiencies? This is the area that most businesses dislike addressing, because no one likes to consider negative things and it might be necessary to completely rethink a project that a great deal of time has been spent on. It is therefore very important for you to be honest. The sooner you resolve the problems you have identified, the faster your business will function efficiently.

The list you create will by no means be exhaustive but will start to put your findings into some sort of coherent order.

Opportunities

These are factors that may present themselves which are external to your business and are the areas you can exploit to your benefit.

This is why it is necessary to go out and make a physical assessment of your location. For example, a new sports club may be opening and you might be able to advertise in it or even run a clinic from there.

You do need to be aware of windows of opportunity. Will the opportunity presented to you be available for some time or are you dealing with a very short window of opportunity? For example it may be possible for you to get a grant to help to start up your new business, but this particular grant application is only available for the next month. In this case you would want to fill in and send of the application as fast as possible.

Do remember that your competitors are not without their limitations. Try to view their clinic from the perspective of a patient as well as from a professional standpoint and see where their weaknesses might lie.

Do not feel intimidated by being newly qualified. It may actually give you an advantage over an established practitioner, since your studies are fresh in your mind and you may have newer and more effective methods of treating patients.

Threats

Like opportunities, these are external factors which are beyond your control, but you may be able to do something that makes them less of a problem, by acting quickly and intelligently on your analysis. Listing the threats will also make you aware of problems before they arise and will prevent complacency when your business is up and running.

Competition is always a potential threat, but how much of a threat? This is what your analysis should tell you. For example, another practitioner has decided to open up in almost the same area. By performing a SWOT analysis you may decide that, on balance, the major difference between the two of you is location, but your location provides more passing trade, so you decide that you have the advantage and decide to stay where you are.

Like weakness this is always another unpopular area to consider, but if the external threats are not addressed you may find your business in trouble before you have even got it off the ground. Assessing threats will also allow you to develop contingency plans should you need them in the future.

If your competitors are more experienced than you, then try to learn what makes them successful. Is it due to price, quality of treatment, the hours they work, convenient location or the good reputation they have gained? You may have to go out to do some more research, but this is why you perform an analysis. You may not have the answers all at once and may need to refine your research.

Do not forget to look at indirect threats, which are therapists who do not use your chosen therapy, but may be treating similar patients.

The research you do may not be first hand and is therefore 'perceived' from your observations, so be careful to keep your SWOT analysis as objective as possible. Starting up on your own is a very personal undertaking because you are the one at the end of the day to make all the decisions. Try at all times when making choices to keep some emotional distance. The SWOT analysis is a tool to focus your thinking process and give you some guide, but do not entirely rely on it for major decision making.

In order to use it as effectively as possible:

- *Be as realistic as possible.* Wishful thinking can sometimes increase your strengths and decrease your weaknesses.
- *Use specific headings.* Bullet points keep you focused.
- *Always perform your analysis in relation to your competition.* This will give you a reference point for your strengths and weaknesses.
- *Always keep the analysis simple and short.* It is only to give you some direction.
- *SWOT is subjective.* No matter how hard you try there will always be some element of subjectivity, and someone else may well come up with an entirely different analysis because she will have a different viewpoint.

Generally it does not matter where you start in the analysis.

Example of SWOT analysis

Imagine that a newly qualified acupuncturist wants to work from a multidisciplinary clinic. She is able to use a room on a licence and there is a central receptionist to take bookings. A SWOT analysis is shown in Box 11.1. It is not definitive but highlights some of the points the acupuncturist might want to think about.

Strengths

These speak for themselves, but are important and positive points to recognize about working in this situation.

Weaknesses

The downside to working this way is not necessarily a major problem.

A recently qualified practitioner may have an entirely fresh approach to a problem. Experience will eventually be acquired and attendance of postgraduate seminars will enhance work experience.

The receptionist can be educated by the practitioner, either by receiving free treatment or by the practitioner taking time to explain exactly what she does and how she would like her calls taken. Patients' telephone numbers can be taken and called back when the acupuncturist is free.

There is not much the acupuncturist can do about sharing the room, but as this is a relatively risk-free way of renting space it should be considered a minor inconvenience.

Box 11.1

Example of a SWOT analysis for a newly qualified acupuncturist working from a multidisciplinary clinic

STRENGTHS	WEAKNESSES
• Recently qualified New ideas • Good position • Reasonable rent • Good patient exposure to therapy • Receptionist	• Recently qualified, there fore lack of experience • Receptionist may not understand therapy • Will have to share room with other practitioners
OPPORTUNITIES	**THREATS**
• Possibilities of networking • Possibilities of sharing costs of advertising ventures • Other practitioners may refer • Information sharing	• Other practitioners in building • Experience and reputation of other practitioners

Opportunities

Cost sharing is a very positive aspect of this sort of arrangement, providing all the practitioners are amenable, since together they can afford a much larger advertisement than they could pay for individually. Joint advertising can be a very good way of presenting an impressive and unified organization.

Threats

Other practitioners in the building can be a problem and it may be best to have a room share in a clinic where there is no duplication of practitioners, unless the practitioner is particularly successful, in which case the association would be professionally beneficial.

Threats can be turned into opportunities, and the possibilities of networking for patients and information sharing can pay dividends when an association works well.

Political (and legal), economic, sociocultural and technological (PEST) analysis

This allows you to get a wider appreciation of the world outside the confines of your clinic.

Your clinic does not operate in a vacuum and is very much subject to outside forces over which you have no control. It is how you deal with the changes that occur that is important.

Political (and legal) factors

Decisions made by the government eventually have an impact on the everyday running of your practice. Not only is the economy affected but also various aspects of new legislation might require you to make changes to employment contracts or health and safety procedures, which may directly or indirectly affect you financially.

Politics and the decisions politicians make depend on the economy and cultural changes, which may ultimately affect the number of patients going through your clinic. For example a decline in the economy will mean that people will spend less and will only want treatment if it is absolutely necessary.

What new legislation is coming into force? How will this affect the way you work? It may create limitations, thereby making you unable to successfully treat conditions, or it may stop you working entirely, because you do not conform to its requirements.

New legislation may also require you to make alterations to your clinic or the way you work, so this financial burden will have to be considered.

For example, the Disability Discrimination Act 1995 meant that many businesses did not have sufficient wheelchair access and therefore were required by law to improve their premises. These financial considerations will change the budget of a clinic.

If a local health authority funds you, would a change in government affect your provision of treatment? If you intend to have a practice that is very reliant on this funding, then it would be a big financial problem if the funding were to be withdrawn.

Political decisions affect the economy, so it is worthwhile even if you do not have a great interest in the subject to at least have a rudimentary idea of how these decisions can affect you as a practitioner.

Because there are continuous changes taking place, do you need a contingency fund to tide you over?

Economic factors

An appreciation of economic growth or depression will allow you to decide whether to expand or stay as you are. These are often difficult to judge, but high street spending does give a general idea of how relaxed the general public feel about spending their money.

Interest rates. When these go down people will have more money to spend; when they go up they will have less.

High unemployment. This will also affect the amount of money people will have available for your treatment. This would be a consideration in choosing to situate your clinic in an area of high unemployment.

Climate changes. These can dramatically affect the economy. For example, there are areas in the last few years that are subject to repeated flooding and others that have experienced devastating flash floods. This has a local or further-reaching effect, affecting economies that might be reliant on goods from those areas. The effect of the flooding might, therefore, be short term or long term as far as a negative effect on the economy is concerned.

Sociocultural factors

What sort of hours are people working? Some patients may only be able to visit you after work, as some companies may not let them come out during the day, or they may have to work long hours away from home.

This will have an impact on your patient load in normal working hours. To compensate for this, your hours will have to change to accommodate the situation, or you may choose to site your clinic somewhere else, so that you can work during the day.

Technological factors

Cause of seeking treatment. Technology is unlikely to be a threat to the complementary field. In fact, because of technology, many people are now working in high-pressure situations in front of computer screens all day, or from home. This leaves little time for relaxation, and may induce them to seek a form of treatment to relieve their musculoskeletal conditions or improve their well-being.

Method of communicating with patients. Many practitioners have websites, and more people have access to the Internet and are using it to find local services and goods. A well-constructed website encourages patients to ring up and speak to you or communicate via email. This can be a cost-effective way of having permanent advertising with a medium that is being used more frequently.

Methods of staying in touch with patients. Mobile phones allow a practitioner enormous flexibility, with divert services available from landlines. Patients are now starting to book appointments by texting.

Example of PEST analysis

The acupuncturist, having looked at the factors immediately affecting her business, now wants to take a wider viewpoint, so proceeds with a PEST analysis (Box 11.2).

Box 11.2

Example of a PEST analysis for a newly qualified acupuncturist working from a multidisciplinary clinic

POLITICAL	**ECONOMIC**
• New registration system due 2009 • Government grants currently available for small businesses – next month	• Area in process of growth • Executive housing being built locally • Increasing interest rate
SOCIAL	**TECHNOLOGICAL**
• More health awareness • More stress at work	• More people on Internet – website • Mobile phone for easy contact

Political

Fortunately for the acupuncturist, because she does not employ staff or own the building, there is a large amount of legislation which she does not need to worry about.

She has, however, made a note of the new registration system currently under discussion, which should improve the status of acupuncturists in the same way it has for chiropractors and osteopaths.

She has also found information on some government grants that are available, but she will have to apply for them quickly as there is a very limited window of opportunity.

Economic

The area is in economic growth, with new executive housing being prominent. The interest rates nationwide seem to be on the rise, so she may well choose to build up her practice where she is for the moment until she can see where the economy is going.

Social

Even if the economy is not picking up rapidly, people are generally more aware of the value of their health, and with more stress at work there is potential for patients who will need treatment to keep them healthy and at work.

Technological

She has decided to harness new technology and investigate the use of a website. She does have the use of the reception staff at the clinic, but as a sole practitioner, patients may need to contact her when she is not there. Giving a mobile phone number will enable the patients to have a link to their practitioner if they have a query, thus enhancing the practitioner–patient relationship.

Preparing your analysis for use

You have now gathered information about your working environment and analysed it. It has given you an idea of:

- Whether you are going about setting up your business in the right way.
- What adjustments are needed to make your vision work.
- Where you fit into the community.

Now you need to consider your clinic in terms of how you are going to get the patient to it.

Marketing mix

This is the combination of factors that affect patient willingness to come to you for treatment. There are generally seven defined aspects, which consist of:

- *Product.* The therapy you are going to use and whether what you are going to offer will work. This is effectively you and the time you have to perform this task. Apart from the cost of your education to get this far, this is very cost-effective.
- *Price.* What price are you going to be able to charge? This will be covered in Chapter 16 on financial considerations for your business plan.
- *Place.* Where you are going to work. Is it convenient to get to?
- *Promotion.* The methods you will use for making people aware of your services, e.g. advertising. If you have not communicated properly to your potential patients through the mediums you have chosen, then you will have wasted time and money. Your assessment of the most effective promotion may range in cost to your time (e.g. writing an article for a magazine or newspaper), to the costly exercise of a newspaper or journal advertisement.
- *People.* This is not only the person delivering the treatment, but also the person answering the phone. Potential patients will be strongly influenced by the manner in which they are dealt with at this first point of contact. Costs will range from that of an answering machine

to the expense of a good-quality receptionist who knows how to deal with people.

- *Process.* This is the customer experience once they have been to see you. All the marketing you have done will be useless if the patient has not had a positive experience.
- *Physical evidence.* This is the appearance of the clinic and the people within the clinic. This is where redecoration cost comes in. You will have to decide what should realistically be spent to get the clinic looking professional.

Conclusion

Added to the SWOT and PEST analyses, the consideration of the marketing mix is very much the culmination of all your research. From the combination of these three you will start to get a feel for whether the plan you have in mind for your business is a sensible one and they will give you an idea of how to promote your business.

The analyses are really derived from common sense and parts of the process of decision making you may perform on a smaller scale every day. These types of analyses merely provide a formalization of these thought processes.

Although it is not necessary to use PEST or SWOT analyses or the marketing mix verbatim in your business plan, elements of them will come through. Not only are they quick and easy considerations, they are also a useful reference when discussing your business with your lenders, and can be performed quickly at intervals to keep up with the changes around you.

There are more ways of analysing your business than the methods described above, but for practitioners starting their own practice for the first time, a few useful tools are less confusing to work with than an overwhelming variety.

No matter how well established your business becomes, the situations around will constantly change. To ignore them may mean that you will be unable to anticipate a problematical situation which might ultimately affect you financially. Do not, however, look upon these changes as hurdles to cross, but as opportunities, and systematic analysis will enable you to make sense of a large volume of facts and use them to your advantage.

Introduction to advertising and public relations

12

Chapter contents

Advertising and public relations are both means of bringing patients into your clinic, and the two areas can overlap and work together. In order to do this properly their distinct qualities need to be clearly understood.

Clearing up the confusion between advertising and public relations (PR)

Advertising is the most direct way you have of letting people know you have a service to offer them. Mostly you will be required to pay for it, but as a consequence, you will have control over what goes in it. You will also know when the advertisement is to be displayed or published and for what length of time.

Public relations is about getting free and positive publicity for your clinic and requires you to develop working relationships with the patient directly or with people who can influence the patient's decision. This may be in the form of a press release taken up as an item of interest by a newspaper, magazine, radio or television station. PR is also an activity which takes place everyday within your clinic, from the way the telephone is answered to your treatment of a patient.

Examining advertisements placed by practitioners it is easy to see that many people confuse advertising with public relations. They spoil the impact of an advertisement by covering it in small writing that amounts to an editorial.

Generally, advertising lacks subtlety and the effect on the patient should be immediate. Advertising is used to draw the eye towards it and entice the potential patient to register your presence and make contact. You then need to use your PR skills to bring the patient right into your clinic for treatment. Public relations is far more subtle than advertising, more long term in its approach than advertising, and requiring a great deal of investment in personal time.

These distinctions do not mean that there cannot be a natural blurring of boundaries where the two entities can complement each other. For example a website is a form of advertising, but because of its construction can also be an exercise in PR. After you have initially captured your potential patients' attention they can be encouraged by intelligent site construction to browse through the site to read on and learn more about you.

Largely, however, it is important to be aware of the differences so that you use the two mediums to their best advantage.

The main differences between advertising and PR

- *Credibility.* Many practitioners look upon their advertisement as a PR tool, filling it with all sorts of information about themselves and unnecessary details of the treatments they offer. Unfortunately, because it is recognizable as an advertisement, many potential patients may not appreciate this over-the-top effort at trying to sell yourself.
- *An article, which is a form of PR, is often written by a third party or by a practitioner.* It usually has a theme, which is usually an approach to treating a particular condition, or something seen as newsworthy and of interest to the general public. For this reason it is perceived differently from the 'hard sell' of an advertisement and can be seen as an 'endorsement' of that treatment or person by the media.
- *Creative control.* Paying for an advertisement ensures complete control in its content and presentation, so you know exactly what is going to be published. With PR, the final representation of you and your treatment is less predictable.
- *Getting your service out to your market.* You can get your advertising published wherever and whenever you wish, providing it suits your budget. PR cannot be as precisely controlled, as you are at the whim of whoever is giving you or your profession the publicity, particularly if you are pursuing PR from a radio or television station. You not only have to be very astute but also very lucky, since their priority of valuable news changes from day to day and something you have set up weeks in advance can be cancelled or overshadowed by a more newsworthy event.
- *Exposure to the public.* Advertising ensures limited personal exposure to the public, but PR does not. If you decide to involve yourself in PR then you may find you are called upon at frequent intervals to make a

comment. This does raise the public's awareness of you, and makes you more recognizable, but may also bring about more personal exposure than you really want.

- *Writing styles differ.* An advertisement is more immediate, and is laced with brief motivational words to draw patients in. An article produced for the purposes of PR requires an objective discussion of a subject and the attention span of a reader is expected to be much longer than for an advertisement. Articles or appearances on radio or television are not there for you to blatantly sell yourself.

Although there are many clear differences between advertising and PR the two can overlap. It is important, however, to be clear on some of the differentiating aspects of the two, or an advertisement may lose its effectiveness through being an exercise in PR and the PR may seem like an unsubtle push of your services.

Generally your professional association will have someone dealing with PR for you, but you may be asked to act as a spokesperson. It can also take a much simpler form, such as talking to people you meet about what you do. It is certainly always present in your professional relationship with your patient.

If you are unclear on any aspect of advertising or PR, make a list of your queries and ring your professional association for clarification. Someone there should be able to give you clear advice, so that you do not suddenly find you have said or written something that is either inaccurate or inappropriate.

Advertising and promotion

13

Chapter contents

Where can you place advertisements?

Placement, along with appearance, is a very important factor affecting the impact your advertisement will have.

Telephone books

The general consensus within the complementary professions is that telephone books specifically published for business such as the *Yellow Pages* are a very productive form of advertising. Each therapy tends to be included under a specific heading.

Yellow Pages

Corporate advertising. Within the *Yellow Pages* there is a further opportunity to raise your profile with corporate advertising if the publishers have an agreement with your professional body. This is a particularly effective way of advertising in several ways.

- *There is very little effort required to be part of an advertisement that is very professional in appearance.* Several members of a particular professional body can mutually agree to set up a block advertisement and share the cost. One person would have to take sole responsibility for the contract, not only to set it up but also to pay for it, requiring the money to be recouped from the rest of the practitioners advertising in that block.

- *Your status as a professional is enhanced.* The personal advertisement you have placed within the section can be cross-referenced against the corporate advertisement to satisfy the potential patient that you are properly qualified.
- *The cost of being present in a large eye-catching advertisement is reasonable.* This works particularly in your favour, as the corporate rate is a flat rate regardless of how few practitioners are present within the advertisement.

There are a few disadvantages.

- *You will be limited on amount and content.* This is both in terms of size of entry and other qualifications from other therapies.
- *You may not be easy to see.* There may be several entries in the corporate box, swamping your entry. The entries are rotated each year to try to give everyone a chance to be first.

Thomson Local

This concentrates on the local area, by listing helpful telephone numbers such as emergency, business and employment, environment and conservation and local helplines.

Although not currently as popular as the *Yellow Pages*, and covering a smaller geographical area, many people do use it. Because of its size it is easier to pick up and look through compared to the *Yellow Pages* and *The Phone Book*, and appeals to many people because it concentrates on the area where they live or work.

The fact that few businesses advertise with more than a line entry has been seen by many businesses as an opportunity to still make an impact with a relatively small, but well-put-together advertisement.

The Phone Book

The Phone Book is currently underused, as it is relatively new, and like the *Thomson Local* it is seen as a chance to get noticed.

Interestingly, the origins of the *Yellow Pages* were in the classified section of *The Phone Book*. This is now being revived, and the classified section can now be found at the front of *The Phone Book*. Each year has seen an enlargement of the section and, as it is an integral part of *The Phone Book*, potential patients may be more inclined to find a practitioner in it, than bother to find another book. The sections are arranged under alphabetical headings, the same way as in the *Yellow Pages*.

Other publications

Newspapers and magazines

Advertising in newspapers has a very short life. Most newspapers are disposed off within days.

Glossy magazines tend to be kept for a longer period of time and read more than once, so the possibility of your advertisement being seen is greater, as is the price of placing an advertisement. You must also bear in mind that the larger the circulation, the more practitioners you will be competing with. On a national scale you may only be able to afford a small, classified advertisement towards the back of the magazine, when first starting out.

Local magazines featuring events in your county or surrounding area often run special health features. This may enable you to nest your advertisement near an editorial about your particular therapy. You are likely to be advertising near other practitioners, so try to get an idea of what type of practitioner they are and who is writing the editorial. Do not be shy in offering your services, since you are an expert in the area. Quite often the journalist writing the article has a limited knowledge of the subject, and unfortunately you do not have much control over what is written.

Advertising in information booklets for surgeries, hospitals and similar organizations

At intervals, you may receive a call to see if you would like to put advertising in doctors' surgery information booklets, or hospital booklets. Ask to see a sample, and investigate their authenticity by ringing the surgery or hospital the caller claims to represent. Ask for names of other therapists in your professional body who have used the organization in other parts of the country so that you can speak to them to find out if advertising in this way was a worthwhile exercise for them.

Smaller publications

Parish magazines and local residents' publications seem to provide very good returns for a very low budget as they are written with the local community in mind.

General advice

Never be pressed into making split-second decisions on advertising, unless it is something you were thinking of doing anyway in that particular publication.

If you are being asked to make an immediate decision, demand a discount. It is possible that they have genuinely not filled the advertising space and need to fill it as quickly as possible, so you may be able to negotiate.

If you have never heard of the publication, then it is possible that neither has anyone whose attention you wish to attract. If you are considering advertising in a publication that is unknown to you, ask for the name of another practitioner who has used that publication in the past so that you can confirm its credibility.

Display material (posters, business cards, leaflets)

- *Effective posters can catch the attention of passers-by.*
- *They can be placed in a variety of locations.* If they are displayed in places where they will not be noticed or lost amongst other advertisements, they will lose their impact.

- *If you cannot put up the poster yourself go and check to see where it has been placed*, particularly if you are paying for it.
- *Laminated advertisements look very professional and last longer.* Many shops selling office supplies will laminate posters.
- *The advertisement should be changed to match the seasons*, e.g. back problems due to gardening, hay fever in the spring.

Direct mail

This reaches a lot of people directly, but you will have to research who you should send to, so that they are mailed appropriately. The success rate for this type of unsolicited mail is low, probably 1–2%, and unsolicited mail may not be permitted under the code of ethics of your professional body or register.

Once you have an ongoing patient list it is quite acceptable to maintain contact with patients, and they can be asked on their first visit if they would appreciate this service. You may have some interesting news about your treatment you want them to know about, or just want to send a general newsletter.

Some clinics produce a newsletter, but it can be time consuming and difficult to keep up once the clinic becomes busy. If you enjoy journalism, this is a useful way to promote your business, and if you work with an organization, such as sports club, you may be able to attach an article to their newsletter. Sometimes this may be in the form of an e-letter, which will enable you to give a very professional appearance to your article.

Always take care to be accurate and correct in your articles and not to make any unsuitable claims.

Website

More and more people are now using the Internet as a means of accessing information.

- *Many professional bodies will put your name and address on their website.*
- *Your website can be linked to your professional body's website or to sites such as the yell.co.uk website* (see p. 130). In many cases there is a linkage to a map location service allowing the patient to see exactly where you are and print out instructions on how to get to you.
- *Constant maintenance of the website is important.* This does require some attention if current articles are being put on it. If a site is under construction for a long period of time, then this will not inspire confidence.
- *It can be expensive* if you cannot do it yourself, although producing a web page has been made easier and there are now reasonably priced courses (that are tax deductible) run by adult education.
- *When you have a web page the address is on the Internet forever.*
- *Not everyone uses the Internet,* although the exceptions are now likely to be older people who were not brought up with computers. Many people who come to see you may have used it as their first port of call.

Look at other practitioners' websites and see how you feel about them from a patient's point of view.

Key points for an effective website

It may well be that you will hand over the construction and running of your website to a professional company. This area is now highly competitive and therefore you should, with a reasonably uncomplicated website, be able to afford this type of service.

The appearance of the website is merely the tip of the iceberg to the work that needs to go into constructing it.

It is still worth knowing a few points to ensure that you are getting the right service.

- *Keep the site clean and free of clutter.* As with advertisements, keep your words short and sweet to give the site more punch. Dense writing is difficult to read. Break it up into paragraphs of manageable chunks.
- *Keep the look and feel of the site consistent.* The colours and fonts should be standardized. Regardless of which page your potential patients are viewing, they will know they are still on your website.
- *Your home page must open quickly, and should have the clinic title clearly visible.* After this, viewers should not have to click their mouse too many times to reach the part they want to read.
- *Make a simple statement as to what you do.* There must be enough information there to catch the eye and keep your potential patient interested enough to browse the other pages of your site. Also keep your language simple and not too technical.
- *Use just enough images to convey the right information.* Images can slow down the loading of a website, so try to keep the number effective but not so large that your potential patient clicks off the website through boredom. Do not use pictures that might be off-putting to the general public.
- *Navigation buttons should be highly visible and obvious.* Most people want information quickly and do not want to have to hunt for it. If there are a great number of buttons, ensure that a static panel is put at the side of the page so that the main text can be scrolled. This will also mean that the user will not have to keep clicking backwards and forwards to find different pages.
- *Always regularly update information if it is time sensitive.* Out-of-date information will reflect badly on your clinic.
- *Always respond quickly to emails.*
- *Register your website with all major search engines.* Keywords will help search engines find your website more easily. Try to include common misspellings of your keywords.
- *Monitor the search engines* to ensure that they not only locate your site but also give it a high enough ranking when the right keywords are typed in.
- *Ensure the site remains compatible with the latest browser software.*
- *Constant maintenance of the website is required.* This will prevent the content of the website becoming stagnant. Even the complementary profession changes. An out-of-date website does not look professional.

- *Register your domain name*, or someone else may use it. This can be done through Nominet or the National Business Register.
- *Put your website and email address on your business card and your advertisements.*

Within the complementary field it is still not absolutely necessary to have a website, although practitioners that do have them have found their website a useful means of referral.

Although it is possible to construct your own website from templates, to do so and make it appear professional and then maintain it does require dedication and some expertise.

How do you put an advertisement together?

- *Keep it simple and clear.* If possible, use one-word lines or simple phrases. Many people make the mistake of turning the advertisement into a public relations exercise and writing an editorial in a desperate bid to sell themselves to the general public. The majority of people will not take the time to read too much small print unless they are genuinely interested.

  YOU ARE TRYING TO CATCH OTHER PEOPLE'S ATTENTION!

  A short, to-the-point advertisement will look far more professional.
- *If you want to say more, get an editorial.* Try to arrange an editorial with the journal or paper and place it separately, but near to the advertisement. If you have caught your potential patients' attention with the advertisement, then it is likely they will take time to read the editorial.
- *Do not make outrageous claims.* You must not claim to cure diseases, merely treat them. Notifiable diseases, sexually transmitted disease or serious diseases such as cancer cannot be primarily treated by someone who is not a medical doctor, although it is reasonable to treat the patient's well-being.
- *Proofreading is essential.* No matter how professional the advertisement, misspellings and incorrect statements will ruin your professional credibility. You must demand to see a proof before the advertisement is placed. Do not forget that you will be paying for it.

Checklist for effective advertising

- *Your advertising should attract attention.* It should be bold, and easy to read and understand. Use of colour should make it stand out but not look garish. It should be clear and memorable.
- *Your advertising should create interest and should be relevant.* Make sure that the material you use is applicable to the type of patients you are

trying to attract. They need to identify with what you are saying and you should make them feel that you have the answer to their problem.
- *Your advertising should create a desire to make contact with you.* Catching their interest is just the first stage. The advertising now has to make them take the next active step of coming to see you. This is where you will know whether you market research has been thorough, as you have identified the patients' needs.
- *Are the contact details clear and correct on your promotional material?* This is an obvious point, but so often overlooked in the haste to get promotional material out.

Conclusion

Advertising is essential for any business, but does not need to be expensive.

It is very easy to get carried away with offers made on advertising, so bargain hard and do not exceed your budget.

Do not get pressurized into placing an advertisement. Do not forget the advertisers need you more than you need them.

Before embarking on any form of advertising, read your professional code of ethics carefully to make sure that you stay within them. Always check with your professional body if you are not sure.

Useful websites

Australia

http://www.auda.org.au/domains/au-domains/

Australian Domain Name Administrator
Information about registering domain names.

Canada

Many websites are bilingual.

http://www.cira.ca/

Canadian Internet Registration Authority

New Zealand

Governmental websites are bilingual.

http://www.dnc.org.nz/

New Zealand Domain Name Commissionaire

UK

http://www.start.biz/home.htm

National Business Register

http://www.nominet.org.uk

Nominet

Internet registry for .uk domain names.

http://www.yell.co.uk

Yell.co.uk

USA

http://www.nic.us/

NeuStar

US Registry operator for US domain name registration.

Public relations 14

Chapter contents

One of the most vital factors in public relations (PR) is to have information to hand which originates from a reliable background. This is why membership of a reputable professional body is so important and why postgraduate education will keep you well informed as to your profession's current opinion on the approach to treatment.

You never know what form PR can take. It can be as simple as a conversation on the street or communicating with a potential patient who has rung in for information, to appearing on television.

The way you conduct your public relations will define the way you appear to not only your potential patients but also your existing ones, and will have a direct impact on your success as a practitioner. In other words, the way you conduct yourself both outside and inside your clinic is part of your PR.

It is important to remember that you have chosen a profession where it is impossible to hide behind a door, since every treatment you give is an interpersonal interaction.

Out and about

- *Enthusiasm.* One of the most important aspects in this particular area will be the enthusiasm for your work. Money spent on sophisticated advertising will be a complete waste of money if you do not exude visible pleasure from performing your chosen vocation. Enthusiasm is the most infectious form of promotion a patient can be exposed to.
- *Prepare an explanation of your therapy and what it can do.* Self-promotion can be a hurdle for many people to overcome. There is nothing wrong with talking to people you meet about your work, but you must make sure that you have a stock explanation of what it is you do or you will appear to be unsure of yourself. By having a simple, but thorough explanation available you will appear confident and professional.
- *Have professionally printed business cards to hand.* Handing out a well-thought-out and professionally printed business card during your impromptu conversations is a perfectly acceptable way of promoting your business, providing you are not overly aggressive in your approach. If you have a website then it is a good idea to put the address on the card.
- *Contact the local businesses.* This can be done on a very personal level, probably when you shop there. Again, you do not need to be pushy, since complementary therapy is usually a source of interest to most people, and even if shopkeepers may not use you themselves they may consider mentioning you to other people they see while working, if you exude confidence, knowledge and enthusiasm for your work.
- *Use friends and relatives.* If your friends or relatives understand exactly what it is you do and know how to talk to people, they can help in a very time-consuming and labour-intensive activity. It is likely they will be very enthusiastic and you can brief them on how you would like to appear to the general public. Give them your cards to hand out when the opportunity arises. This widens the area you can cover and can help you if you are naturally shy and find it difficult to approach people in this way.

Giving talks

This can be a cost-effective way of meeting the public. At the most it will involve the price of a slide projector and a few slides, along with your time and the cost of petrol or bus fare to get to wherever you have arranged to give the talk.

Practitioners can find themselves giving talks to a range of people, from the level of a self-help group to a group of doctors. Pitch your talk to your audience's interests, and do not make it too technical.

Women's groups are very influential and usually have a wider network than is immediately obvious. Never underestimate the ability of these groups to encourage people to come in to see you. They are usually also a delight to talk to and very interested in what you have to say.

The facilities available to you for your presentation will vary from nothing to equipment for a PowerPoint presentation. Ask what is likely to be available. Slide projectors are relatively inexpensive now that computers have taken over, and you may even be able to pick one up second-hand, so investing in one could prove useful.

If you are not used to speaking in public, then practise on your friends. Knowing your subject well will give you confidence and inspire interest and confidence in your abilities as practitioner.

Here are a few tips:

- *Ask how long you will be given to talk.* This will give you a time span to work to.
- *Arrive in plenty of time to sort things out.* There are always some minor problems with any venue. This time will also allow you to orientate yourself to the layout and help you feel more relaxed.
- *Always try to time your talk.* There is nothing worse than overrunning. Some groups only have a room for a limited time, so make sure you do not overrun.
- *Be prepared to be flexible.* Many groups do not properly start at the time advertised, so allow enough time for stragglers to appear.
- *Be aware of your audience's interest level.* Keep scanning the audience to make sure what you are saying is being taken in and that their attention is not wandering. If you are losing them, you must adapt. It may be that your language it too technical or that you have talked for long enough, so make adjustments, such as reducing the length of your talk or changing pace. This will come with experience.
- *Allow plenty of time for questions.* There are usually plenty of these and sometimes people prefer to talk to you on a one-to-one basis, rather than in front of other people.
- *Demonstrations are well received.* Because of legal constraints, this is not always possible. If you are wary about using someone in the audience then bring someone with you.
- *Bring the tools of your trade.* A chiropractor could bring a demonstration spine. A herbalist can bring packeted herbs for the audience to look at. An aromatherapist can bring the different essential oils. Stimulation of the different senses adds to the experience.

Your talks can be teaching sessions if your therapy lends itself to this type of interaction. For example, an aromatherapist may demonstrate how to mix a combination of oils.

Adult education or open learning class

This is a very useful way of promoting yourself, but it is no longer the relaxed system it was. The teaching sessions are now run as modules with compulsory assessments at the end of the course, or in cases where a craft is being taught, as presentation of a finished piece that the student has made during the course.

Despite the amount of work now required by the lecturer involved, it is still seen as rewarding and may be a course of action for practitioners who like to be part of an educational system.

Articles in newspapers and magazines

Usually newspapers or magazines only publish an article if it is newsworthy. This may involve an unusual treatment or you having gained a certain amount of positive notoriety, for instance treating a celebrity patient, or public recognition for work in your field.

Specialist magazines tend to have an in-house complementary expert. If they do not, then this is a useful opportunity to offer your services.

Free newspapers usually want you to take out some form of advertising in order to warrant an editorial, but do not be afraid to ask whether you can write the editorial.

When writing an article for a newspaper or magazine there are several things to remember:

- Do not use complicated technical terms.
- Use short sentences that are easy to read.
- Be factual, and make sure your statements are not unsubstantiated.
- Make sure you mention your professional body early on in the piece and what their function is.
- Be precise about your use of words.

Writing a press release

Most professional bodies are very experienced at writing press releases, most hiring a PR firm to make contacts and prepare press releases. Before you take it upon yourself to send one out, it would be a good idea to have it checked. This will prevent duplication and will confirm the appropriateness of your subject matter.

Press releases are composed in a particular format, for ease of reading and impact.

- *Always put the release date at the top.*
- *Start with an eye-catching headline.* The psychology is similar to that of an advertisement. You want your audience to read further.
- *Do not forget to put your name or that of your clinic near the beginning.*
- *Say where the story is likely to be of interest.* Is it relevant for your local village or town or the whole county?

- *In as few words as possible say why it is news.*
- *Give an idea of for how long the news is valid.* This may be an announcement of your clinic opening, which is on a specific day. Therefore the news is valid for a limited time.
- *Include an editor's note, with the basic facts about your particular therapy or professional body.* Not everyone will understand the nature of your therapy or how important membership of your professional body is.
- *Make sure you give your name and telephone number.*
- *Keep the release short and interesting.*

Avoid the following with your press release:

- *Writing down the wrong contact name or telephone number.*
- *Addressing it to someone who is no longer at the newspaper, radio or TV station.*
- *Getting the news editor's name right, but using the wrong title.*
- *Sending it too late for someone to do something with it.* For example, sending a press release about your clinic open day after it has happened.
- *Sending it after it has already been published in another newspaper or aired on another radio or TV station.*

The person you will be sending the press release to will receive many press releases a day, so it is important to get the format of the press release and etiquette right to give yours a better chance of being read and acted on.

An example of a press release can be found in the appendix to this chapter (p. 140).

Networking

Networking with other professionals can be counted as a form of PR.

There are many positive aspects to having a network of other professionals you can send your patients to. Patients do appreciate honesty and sending them to other practitioners, who you know are highly competent in their field, is usually perceived as an intelligent referral by a practitioner genuinely interested in their welfare.

There are several elements to networking:

- *It is very important if you are working alone.* It will stop you becoming isolated and may be a useful support if a crisis occurs, e.g. if you are ill and need patients to be seen by someone responsible who will then send them back to you.
- *It provides business opportunities.* You may not be able to perform a certain treatment that the patient needs and, likewise, another therapist may need your assistance. Patients appreciate the care you have taken to ensure a successful outcome for them. Inter-referral with a therapist you trust is a very good way of building up a practice.

- *It does require constant effort on your part to keep contact* and it may take some time for there to be a pay-off, as there has to be a situation of mutual trust and interest in the patient's health for it to work successfully.
- *You may have to offer a discount* such as waiving the initial consultation fee and charging a normal treatment fee instead. This may seem a financially inefficient way to run a business, but the patient and the other therapist will see it as a desire to work together to achieve results, which is positive PR.

It may be worth joining the local Chamber of Commerce. See how active the one is in your area for small businesses. If it is your intention to tap into the firms in the area, then there are always events being held for members that can cost very little or are free. They are designed to allow people to network, giving you an opportunity to give other local businesses an idea of how your services may benefit them. This does require a very outgoing personality, however, and may not suit every practitioner.

Exhibitions

These can vary enormously and you may find yourself displaying by the side of a therapy whose governing body does not require the same educational or ethical standards as your own.

If the exhibition is well run and professional it may be a good way of meeting potential patients face to face, allowing you to sell your treatment.

Do make allowances in your costing for transport, exhibition materials and rental of your space.

Holding open days

These are usually an acceptable way of presenting yourself to the general public. If you are a part of a multidisciplinary clinic that holds this sort of event, it is a good idea to be involved.

- *Open days are a good way to get the public in to see you,* particularly if you are based in a town or city. You may be able to give demonstrations or at least talk to your potential patients.
- *Make sure it is publicized.* There will be no point holding an open day if no one knows about it. Local radio can often be very helpful in announcing this type of event, providing it is a community event.
- *Check this event with your insurance company.* Technically you are covered for public liability, but there may be considerations because of the large volume of people and the fact you have the tools of your trade on display. You may also want to check fire regulations regarding numbers of people.

- *Get people to help you* keep an eye on the clinic contents and look after the welfare of your visitors, while you concentrate on talking to your potential patients. If you have relatives or friends who have a thorough understanding of your therapy, then try to have them with you.
- *Pay attention to security,* things can go missing, and you may have to consider removing such items as computers, since these sorts of occasions can be used to carefully examine the contents and security of a premises in preparation for a burglary. Do check with your insurers to make sure you are adequately covered for the event.

Dealing with the media

If you are called by anyone in the media whom you have no previous experience of, there are several things to consider.

- *Are the issues going to be contentious?* Some programmes or newspapers are notorious for encouraging confrontation.
- *Who else is going to be involved?* In some cases you may be facing someone who is known for a strident opposite viewpoint.
- *Is the programme going out live?* Editing can change the most innocent of statements into something quite different. If the programme is live, then mistakes cannot be covered up.
- *Do you thoroughly understand the issues that will be discussed?* There is nothing worse than stumbling for an answer or making inappropriate comments because you do not fully comprehend the nature of the discussion.
- *Do not give advice that could lead to litigation.* For example it is not appropriate to give a diagnosis after a brief discussion with a listener or viewer. You can talk around the subject and this will enable you to reiterate the importance of consulting a qualified practitioner who is a member of a recognized body.

You will have to be careful not to be seen to be actively endorsing any particular products.

It is more than likely that there will be people involved in your association who are experienced in media matters and will provide you with useful information. If you feel that exposure to the media is beyond your capabilities, ask the association if there is someone who can get involved instead of you.

Dealing with negative publicity

It is to be hoped that you will not have to deal with this on a personal basis, but it may well be that something unfortunate has occurred to a patient who has been treated by another therapist, or that a negative piece of research has raised local media interest. Whatever the reason for the bad news, it is important to do several things:

- *Be proactive in dealing with the issue.*
- *Find out all the details surrounding the news so that you are fully informed.* There is nothing worse than dealing with any item of news, good or bad, with only half the information. Getting the facts wrong will ruin your credibility.
- *Consult with your professional body.* Any interview you give or comment you make should tally with the views of your professional body. They should have someone you can consult who will be conversant with how to handle the situation, so do not make any statement or give an interview until you have spoken to them. Take the name and number of the journalist if you are contacted, then call back as quickly as possible once you have taken advice.
- *Be truthful.* Fabrications are usually found out since they rarely stand up to scrutiny.
- *Be calm and factual.* Do not become emotional no matter how impassioned you feel about the subject.
- *Negative publicity can frequently be turned into positive publicity.* The way in which negative publicity is usually presented is so that it grabs the public's attention. This is why you need all the facts and someone to help to make some sense of the situation.

Logos

It is important to have a logo. There are so many copyright-free images available that it is easy to add a professional touch to your stationery and business cards. Computers now make the process of design very simple so you can easily design your own.

Do give careful thought to the image you use, as this will become synonymous with you and your clinic.

In looking for or designing a logo there are a few simple rules to follow:

- *Your logo should reflect the nature of your therapy.* For example, many acupuncturists use a yin yang symbol, chiropractors use a derivation of a spine, herbalists use a floral design.
- *Do not use too much detail.* A simple logo is much more recognizable than a complex one and is much more easily produced.
- *The logo should be reproducible in any size.* Try enlarging it to poster size and see if it looks untidy or loses impact.
- *Make sure it looks good in black and white.* This will highlight just how well defined your logo is. If it is not effective in black and white, then its reproduction in another colour will not be effective.

Why membership of a professional body is helpful with your PR

- *Belonging to a professional organization gives you credibility.*
- *They will be proactive nationwide on your behalf with radio, TV and magazine slots.* Most professional bodies hire PR companies who work hard on your behalf to encourage the media to write articles or bring practitioners on to their programmes.
- *They can save you the cost of producing leaflets,* as there will be a space on the back of theirs to put your name and address stamp.
- *You can put your address and details on their website.*
- *Corporate advertising.* Membership of a professional body may allow you to take part in corporate advertising and there may be other cases when group advertising will be possible.
- *Networking with other therapists in your association may be possible.*
- *They will give you advice on PR.*
- *Patients may have already experienced treatment from someone in your organization and therefore know what to expect.*
- *Patients can compare prices between you and other members of your association.*

Conclusion

Like advertising, PR can be very visible, but its approach is much more subtle.

PR is not something you can perform once and walk away from. It is an ongoing process that requires time and effort, but may cost you very little financial outlay.

It will be, over the years, one of the key factors to play a role in bringing patients into your clinic and retaining them on your lists.

Appendix

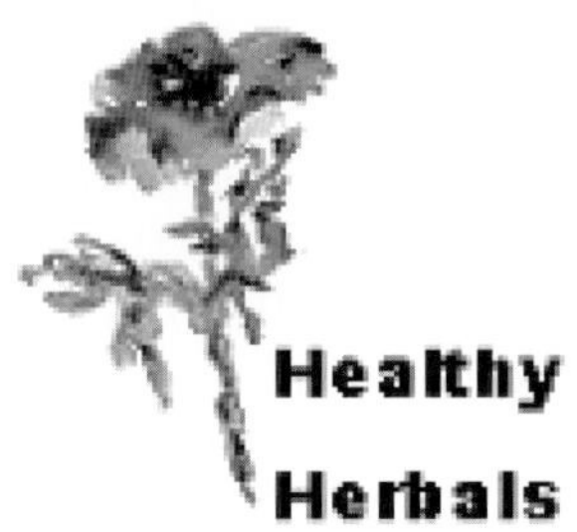

15th February 2005

Celebrity gardener's career rescued by herbs – TV gardener Hortense Petunia returns triumphantly to our screens –

TV gardener and national institution Hortense Petunia was last night back in front of the cameras after six weeks' absence. Her debilitating condition? Hay fever.

'It was a problem I'd never experienced before. Having worked most of my life outdoors, I was shocked by the severity of the condition and that I could experience something I thought wouldn't affect someone of my age group. I couldn't even go out into my own garden without my nose running profusely and my eyes streaming. As you can imagine going on camera looking red eyed and constantly blowing my nose was an impossible situation to be in. Nothing seemed to work and the medication I was taking made me want to sleep all the time. My career and my life's work seemed at an end.'

Fortunately Miss Petunia was quickly directed towards herbal treatment by a friend who had been treated at the Healthy Herbals Clinic. She had this to say about her experience.

'My friend had been extolling the virtues of herbal medicine for years, but I had not paid much attention to what she had said. I was amazed to find how thorough Greta Hanson of Healthy Herbals was, taking a full medical history and performing a thorough medical examination. Not only did I receive herbal medicine but was given all sorts of useful advice on food and supplements. I have to say I now feel better than I have done for years.'

Pollen count levels have been rising steadily over the last few years to an all-time high in June this year. An estimated 12 million people suffer from red eyes, runny noses and headaches in the hay fever season. The National Pollen Research Unit has forecast that pollen counts will start falling to normal levels over the next two to three weeks, but could still reach peaks in July.

Dr Frederick Arbour, consultant physician in rhinology, allergy and immunology at the National Throat, Nose and Ear Hospital in Anytown, said: 'People who have never suffered hay fever before are starting to experience symptoms, sometimes to the point of serious debilitation.'

The Countrywide weather centre has warned that pollen counts over the next few weeks are expected to remain high.

Greta Hanson, a member of the Countrywide Herbal Association and proprietor of Healthy Herbals comments: 'I have seen a marked increase in people suffering from the effects of hay fever in the last few months. It now seems to be affecting a much broader age range than before. Herbal medicine is a gentle and effective way to treat any age group for this type of condition, but being a herbalist is not just about treating the problem but looking at the well-being of the person. This will include nutritional advice as well as working with the patient on general lifestyle issues.'

To find out more information about the Countrywide Herbal Association (CHA) visit www.cha.co.uk or call 0111 178908.

Or call: Greta Hanson at Healthy Herbals: 03333 678993.

Healthy Herbal Press Enquiries

Greta Hanson
Tel: 03333 678993
Email: ghanson@pelican.com

Notes to Editors

CHA herbalists see hundreds of patients each day and are able to provide a safe and effective form of treatment to every age group.

The CHA represents well over 80% of the country's herbalists, with over 700 members. Every member of the CHA has to abide by a strict code of ethics and follows a well-defined dispensary code of practice. The association will only accept graduates who have trained for at least three years at a recognized college.

Herbal medicine is not purely symptom orientated but seeks to discover any underlying health problem and treat each person as an individual.

Herbalists treat a wide range of acute and chronic conditions and members of the CHA will take a full medical history and consider the medication regime of each patient before prescribing a combination of herbs specifically for that patient.

To find out more information about the CHA please visit www.cha.co.uk or call 0111 178908.

Part 3

Financial matters

Finance introduction 15

Chapter contents

This is the area that causes complementary practitioners the most anguish and is something that many try to brush to one side, hoping it will go away. It is, however, something that will be a very important part of your working life. If you have reached the point of looking at your finances, then you may well have dealt with the complex aspects of marketing. Like marketing, dealing with the financial aspects of your clinic only requires a little dedication, methodical application and practice.

Keeping your accounts

When you are first starting out, your accounts should be very simple to keep, requiring only a standard accounts ledger or spreadsheet. Computerized professional accounting packages are available, and if you do decide to opt for one, it will not need to be expensive, since your incomings and outgoing will be very simple.

Some accountants feel, however, that in the hands of the inexperienced, these packages can cause an immense amount of problems. It only takes one entry to cause a myriad of miscalculations that may take some time to trace, whereas the same mistake in a written ledger is much easier to locate. So if you choose to use a computer package, do make sure you are very conversant with it.

It does get a little more complicated when you take on an employee; even so, computer packages are available that help you to work out an employee's pay, and HM Revenue & Customs can be very helpful with queries.

Your tax return

It is possible to do a self-assessment form for HM Revenue & Customs and they offer free advice to help you fill it out. Your time is money, however, and the time you spend on your tax form may be consuming valuable clinic or quality personal time. It is also possible you may end up paying more tax than you should, so unless you have a financial background it is better to get an accountant to do the work for you.

Accountants charge according to seniority, type of work, and expenses, and usually per hour, so before you engage one it is a good idea to specify in writing exactly what it is you want done for you and ask what the charge is likely to be. Make it clear that you are self-employed. It is better to have an accountant who is conversant with the complexities of being self-employed.

The bill you will receive from your accountant should be itemized according to the work you have agreed between you, e.g. preparing a tax return, or providing advice. The more thorough you are with your book-keeping, the less work an accountant will have to do, thus saving you money.

The accounting year

This is a 12-month period running from when you first start your business, and does not have to run from the beginning of the tax year. You will be asked to pay tax twice a year, currently in January and July.

Unfortunately, tax for the self-employed is calculated in advance, so if you have a very good year, your next year's tax will be high. This means that you will have to put money aside if the next year is not as profitable, so that you will have adequate funds to pay your tax bill. Tax can only be claimed back by a readjustment when you next have to pay tax, but a good accountant will negotiate on your behalf to get your tax bill reduced before you pay it.

Allowable expenses

An allowable expense is defined as any expense that is necessary for your business to function. It must be for the exclusive use of the business, but some items can be allowed if a percentage of their use is for the business, e.g. telephone, electricity, car, etc.

Premises costs. These will include rent, business rates, utilities and repairs or alterations carried out.

If you are working from home, ask your accountant for a sensible annual flat rate that can be charged by you to your business. It is possible to charge for a percentage of the rates or mortgage, but this tends to complicate the picture, as your home may then be liable for business rates or capital gains when you come to sell your house. Again, it is best to ask your accountant's advice.

Employee costs. These include wages/salaries, pensions, insurances and employees' National Insurance (NI) contributions.

If you do choose to pay your receptionist in cash make sure you have deducted the correct amount of PAYE and NI contributions. Make sure that the transaction is carefully documented with your employee's signature against the amount.

Paying by cheque leaves a clear record that you have paid your employee and exactly how much.

Ensure you have the P45 form from your employee's last job, or if you do not then you must fill in form P46.

Stock. These are thing that you sell such as herbs, vitamins, pillows, etc.

Services. This includes people you have to call in for maintenance or repairs, e.g. plumbers.

Motor expenses. These are repairs on your car, servicing, petrol, road fund licence, etc.

Travel/subsistence. These are expenses you incur when working away from your usual premises or when on a course, and will include such things as hotel bills and food.

Marketing and advertising. Money has to be set aside for some advertising or PR activity. You will undoubtedly use some for directory advertising such as in the *Yellow Pages*.

Bad debts. Occasionally you may have patients who receive treatment and for one reason or another have no means of paying at the time. On the whole, patients are fairly honest and will get the money to you somehow. If they incur a bad debt, which has not been paid in a reasonable amount of time, you can pursue them in the small claims court. More often than not this is expensive in terms of time away from your clinic and expenses incurred, so writing off the debt may be the best solution.

Do not put a patient on account unless the person is known by you to be reliable. Many large healthcare companies are billed by practitioners and are usually very reliable and punctual in their payments.

Finance. Bank charges and interest on loans, hire purchase or lease can be written off against tax.

Depreciation. This will occur on your car and equipment over a period of time.

Miscellaneous. These are items such as travelling costs, petrol, hotels, training costs incurred after business has been started, stationery, postage, professional services, e.g. accountants, solicitors, and various insurances.

Non-allowable expenses

Entertaining. Entertaining someone other than staff is not an allowable expense; therefore clinic events that include partners and families cannot be deducted against tax.

Clothing. Only clothing that cannot be worn for anything but your job will be allowed, e.g. clinic jackets.

Depreciation. You may, however, claim capital allowances in respect to the purchase of equipment.

Fines. E.g. parking tickets, speeding fines.

Miscellaneous items of tax information

Below a certain income, which will change from time to time, you will not be required to pay tax. If this is the case, you will not be able to claim business expenses against tax, and will be leading a very meagre existence.

It is possible for a person to be in employment and self-employed, for example you may run your own clinic, but also teach. This is where your accountant will be useful to untangle the complications of this way of working.

Registering for tax

You must apply to be registered as a self-employed person within 3 months of starting work. A form for this purpose is available online (see p. 152).

Exemptions from National Insurance

You will be exempt from paying National Insurance if:

- You are sick for a prolonged period of time.
- You have a maternity allowance.
- You have reached a pensionable age.
- Your earnings are below a certain limit for that year.

Again it has to be stressed that most of these situations, unless you have a lifestyle that matches this lack of income, will place you in severe financial stress.

Value added tax (VAT)

Registered professionals such as chiropractors and osteopaths are exempt from VAT. Other complementary professions are not.

The level of turnover above which you will have to pay VAT varies every year. This threshold level is fairly high and it is most unlikely you will need to register immediately, but your accountant will be able to advise you on this matter.

If you are registered for VAT your invoice should show the following:

- Your business name and address.
- Your VAT registration number.
- Your invoice number.
- The date of the invoice or the date of supply, or the date of receipt of payment (tax point).
- What the invoice is for.
- Amount of treatments or goods supplied and percentage of VAT.
- Cost of each treatment or goods.
- The amount and rate of VAT on each item.
- Any discounts that were given.
- The total cost excluding VAT.
- The separate VAT cost.
- The total including VAT.

This tax invoice is not usually necessary for treatments and supply to patients, unless they want one.

It is best to be registered to pay per quarter.

Fortunately by being paid cash on each visit you will only pay VAT on the money you have taken into the practice, and you will not be required to pay in advance for services you have provided.

Pre-trading cost. This needs to be checked with an accountant, but some books used on your course may be allowable, as are the setting-up costs.

Alterations to your home may not be allowable if you have not worked in some capacity there before, so again check.

Financial record keeping

It is very important to do this properly and keep on top of it. If you are self-employed you will need to keep your records for 5 years, and if a limited company or in partnership, for 6 years.

The records you will need to keep are:

- *Cash and cheque payments, etc.* from patients and other sources.
- *Expenditure.* This may be anything from equipment to soap.

- *Petty cash.* If you have a small and separate fund that can be accessed by staff for small items, such as tea and coffee.
- *Drawings.* This is money taken out of the business for your personal use.

All this information will be needed if you are to create a *profit and loss account*.

There are several reasons to keep good records:

- *They provide vital information on how your business is performing.*
- *They enable you to see quickly if you are making a profit or loss.* This allows you to change your spending to adapt to any problems taking place. It will also allow you to plan ahead.
- *They are important for getting mortgages, life insurance, pensions, and further loans.* Most lenders will need to see 3 years of accounts.
- *They help your accountant to reconcile your accounts more easily.* This will ensure that you do not overpay tax, as calculations can be made in plenty of time. The more bookwork you do the less time the accountant will have to spend on your behalf and the lower the fees.

Documentation

Daily takings sheet. This can either be done in the appointment book or on a separate sheet. This way you have an exact record of how much you have taken, as the complementary field is largely a cash business.

Pay-in books and cheque books. These are two very important documents since they will show just how much is going in and out of your business.

Credit card statements. Many practitioners use credit cards as a convenient way of paying wholesalers and use the credit card statement as a means of keeping a tight check on spending, since cash is more difficult to keep track of.

Invoices. These should be kept in a file, usually in order of date, with a note of when they were paid.

Bank statements. These are vital for the running of the business as they enable you to see whether cheques have been presented and anticipate money going into or out of the account.

Cash books and computer spreadsheets. You will need some means of recording your information. This can be something as simple as a ledger or a complex software programme. For a very modest clinic a written cash book is more than adequate; otherwise, computerized software is simple and efficient to use. Do ensure, however, if you are using a computer for your accounts that you back up your files on a regular basis.

Banks

Do not assume that your bank manager is an expert in the particular type of finance you want. He may not be conversant with your profession, which is why you will need to be coherent and have all the information at your fingertips. Bank managers will listen and give advice, but many have not actually run a business of their own.

There is not much to choose between the major banks, although it is worth looking at what they can offer you. Do not forget, as a new customer you should be looking at what the banks can offer you and not the other way round. Even rates on loans can be negotiated.

Your advantage over many other businesses is your cash flow. By receiving money immediately from your patients after their treatment, you will be able to pay cash into your account very quickly. Many medical insurance companies favour the BACS (Bankers Automated Clearing Services) system, which allows them to pay directly into your account. From sending your bill to having the money paid into your account may take less than 2 weeks.

Communicating with your bank is important. If you are running into any problems then inform them ahead of time, rather than wait for them to find out. If you need a larger overdraft, tell them as soon as possible why you require the increase and how long you will need it for.

Although there is more flexibility with an overdraft facility, repayment of the money you owe can be demanded at any time.

Conclusion

Although an unpopular area of consideration for a complementary practitioner, finance is very important and cannot be ignored.

Be methodical in your approach and keep your records carefully right down to the smallest receipt.

It is best to engage the services of an accountant before you start trading. Unless you have been an accountant or have an in-depth understanding of the finance and tax system, you are likely to encounter problems.

Useful websites

Australia

http://www.ato.gov.au/

Australian Taxation Office

Canada

Many websites are bilingual.

http://www.cra-arc.gc.ca/
Canadian Revenue Agency

New Zealand

Governmental websites are bilingual.

http://www.ird.govt.nz/
New Zealand Inland Revenue

UK

http://www.hmrc.gov.uk/
HM Revenue & Customs

http://www.hmrc.gov.uk/forms/cwf1.pdf
HM Revenue & Customs
Form for registering as a self-employed person.

USA

http://www.irs.gov/
Internal Revenue Service
US Department of the Treasury.

Financial considerations for your business plan

16

Chapter contents

Now you have a system worked out it is time to start looking at the financial side of your business plan so that you know exactly what budget you will need and how you are going to raise the money for your new venture.

How do I start to work out my financial requirements?

There are two financial areas that have to be considered when preparing your budget:

- Living expenses.
- Business expenses.

Living expenses

These should not cause too much trouble since you should already have a very good idea of how much it costs you to live and you are used to handling your personal finances.

It is very important to itemize these expenses in terms of:

- *Mortgage or rental of property.*
- *Council Tax.*
- *Services.* These are your electricity, gas, water and telephone.
- *Motor.* If you already have a car, then you will need to itemize how much it costs to repair and service a year, and the cost of hire purchase (if there is any) and insurance.
- *Food.* Average out your weekly bills.
- *Clothing.*
- *Recreation.* Cost of holidays, eating out, days out, leisure activities.
- *Sundries.* Anything else not covered by the above.

Is there anyone you could share expenses with, such as a partner, spouse or tenant?

As well as normal living expenses, you may have the responsibility of a partner or family and need to take out life insurance or permanent healthcare insurance, so that there is some income still available if you are no longer able to earn.

Try to decide truthfully what you are able to live on. There is nothing worse than a bank balance that is out of hand. There is nothing more helpful to you than your bank manager being able to see you have budgeted sensibly.

It is important to be honest about how much you spend or you will exceed your budget and find yourself in financial difficulties.

Business expenses

It would be nice to start with a newly furnished and decorated clinic, but this is not always a possibility. Getting carried away with fixtures and fittings and equipment for a new clinic is a common fault, not only of the complementary professions but also of many businesses newly starting up. This stems from the mistaken belief that only new and expensive decoration will impress patients. The reality is that providing the place is clean, tidy, well maintained and houses a competent and caring practitioner, the patients will be more than happy.

You need to have a clear idea of just how much money you will need to borrow in order to get your business off the ground and earning you a living.

There are two options available to you when you start your clinic:

- *Carry on working in your current job.* This way you are still earning a living wage while you build up your clinic.

- *Give up your current job and live on your savings and loans.* In this case you may need to take out a loan that will sustain you for long enough to make your clinic viable.

You have to be ruthless and spend only the amount you have allotted yourself, with something set aside for emergencies, particularly if you own your own premises.

Costing out every item will allow you to see exactly how much you will be spending. By understanding the financial implications of what you are about to undertake you will be able to see what you really can afford.

How to work out a budget

Business expenses

The thought of doing this is often quite daunting, as many practitioners have had little experience of thinking their way through this type of budget. It is not really too complicated, particularly if you are just starting out, since you will want to start with the simplest set-up that is suitable for you. Working out these expenses is not dissimilar to your household budgeting, and you will already have an idea of the cost of items, such as services, that are common to both budgets.

You have already made a decision on where you want to work, so you have an idea of what equipment you will need and whether you will be paying for wages, services and rent.

Worked examples

These are in appendices at the end of the chapter and have been done to enable you to work through the process of how much money you will ultimately have to earn a year to keep financially viable, then ultimately make a profit. Although figures have been kept as realistic as possible, for simplicity all of the calculations have been made with the idea that the practitioner in the example has a business that will be financially self-sufficient in 2 years.

This time span may be considered optimistic, and the reality may be that it will take a little longer. The calculations, however, are to demonstrate to you how to go about ultimately producing a cash-flow and profit/loss forecast. It was considered much easier to follow the flow of calculations from worked examples than from verbal descriptions and isolated calculations. The examples show that the practitioners had each decided on a certain standard of living, and following these examples you will be able to tailor the process to your own requirements.

The three worked examples are of the usual situations you may find yourself working in. This should help you understand how to go about working out annual costs and how many patients a day will be needed to help you break even. You may choose to work in a mixture of two or all three scenarios, and it is not uncommon for practitioners to do just that. You may also decide that you can manage without certain items such as a receptionist, car, or computer.

The examples assume a 4-day week, but as can be seen from the example of home practice, not many patients are needed to break even, and working in the evening or at the weekend may put you on quite a good financial footing fairly quickly if you do not feel you can give up your current job immediately.

The calculations in the examples are presented in a way that should be self-explanatory.

Calculating a breakdown of fixed costs

It is a good idea to get to grips with your likely expenditure. You can consider your costs in any order. The following is a comprehensive list of items you will need to consider, although there may be other items you might wish to add.

Service charges

These are ongoing charges that you will *not* be able to dispense with.

Wages

Do you need a member of staff? Employees account for a large percentage of the running costs (see the analysis of pie charts calculated from fixed costs, below). It may therefore be useful when you are starting out to see if you can recruit a friend or relative who will help free of charge or for some arrangement other than cash. Tax laws frequently change so it is worth consulting your accountant to find out if there is any tax advantage to any members of your family working for you.

Utilities and council rates

These, like wages, are a fixed cost; in other words they cost the same amount of money regardless of how busy you are. Unlike employees, you have to have them.

Owning property or renting. You are responsible for the utility bill.

Renting a room under licence. Utilities and council rates are included in the cost of the room. Room rental can be a percentage of the takings or a fixed amount.

Note on utilities and local council charges. When taking charge of renting a suite of rooms or a building, all of your services should be metered. Sometimes, however, in older buildings the water may not be metered. The standard water rate on a commercial property is far in excess of that of a domestic property, even though you may be using only the same amount of water as a domestic dwelling. Do check that a water meter is in place and also the amount you will have to pay per quarter for each utility before you take on a property.

If you are working from home, a percentage of the utilities can be charged against the business, but check with your accountant, who will advise you. It may be better, as in the example of the acupuncturist working from home (Appendix 16.1, p. 166), to charge a flat rate to avoid a possible capital gains levy on selling and ongoing business rates.

It may well be that you will be paying business rates to the council and this must be accounted for on top of the basic rent.

Cleaning

Initially you may be able to clean the interior and windows of the building, saving this expense for when you become busier and can afford it.

Safety

If you are renting, the landlord should be responsible for meeting the fire regulations. If this is in dispute, your solicitor will be able to clarify this.

There are certain safety checks with electrically operated goods, such as the kettle, vacuum cleaner, etc., and your specialist equipment such as couches that by law must be carried out.

Alarm system

A fully serviced alarm may be a condition of your business insurance, although it is not always necessary to have permanent coverage to a central monitoring station.

If you are working from home, bear in mind that you will have to tell your patients when you are going away.

Vehicle costs

A new car is not necessary. You may already own a car you have already paid for, or you may not need one. Even a second-hand vehicle can add substantial costs to your budget, and there are always running costs involved.

Insurance

Largely, this amounts to business and car insurance and is a necessary expense. Look around for a good deal that meets all your criteria.

Advertising

The cost of advertising can escalate out of all control. Phone books are probably where you want to spend most of your budget, and for these you can easily get an uncomplicated and immediate quotation. Once established, this form of advertising is a standard expense that will be a routine payment.

If you are going to advertise elsewhere, you must build the cost of repeat advertising into your budget, using written quotations you have been given.

The sudden impulsive urge to advertise, particularly if the offer seems tempting, may send you over budget, so be very rigid in your attitude to expenditure in this area. It is very important to be very clear on exactly what money you are prepared to set aside for this budget and not to exceed it.

Stationery

This is one of the opportunities you have to present a professional image at relatively little cost, so make the most of it.

If you choose to produce your own stationery then choose a good-quality printer with mid-weight, watermarked paper. There is still, however, a certain finesse to professionally printed notepaper, so the expense could be justified.

Business cards should be produced professionally and finished to a high standard. Although only small, their feel and quality is quickly noticed. Get written quotations from several printers and examples of their work.

Compliment slips and receipts are not necessary, since your headed notepaper is multipurpose.

Furniture

If you are working from home you may be able to use the furniture you already have there or borrow furniture.

Second-hand office furniture from office suppliers is also a possibility, so spend some time comparing quality of goods and prices. Buying a group of items may allow you to agree a discount. Do check that there is compliance with health and safety regulations and that the furniture you use is in good repair.

These days, however, new flat-packed furniture can sometimes be bought very cost-effectively from suppliers who are able to buy cheaply and pass the low cost on to the consumer.

Equipment

Professional equipment can be bought second-hand, but do get a specialist firm experienced in servicing the type of equipment you use to give it a safety check before you use it in the treatment of a member of the general public.

It is worth buying a sturdy couch. Although this may increase the cost, it is worth remembering that in your career you will be treating people of all sizes and weights, and a robust couch will last you a long time.

With the advent of the Internet it is now much easier to compare prices of goods to see who has the best deals.

Electrical goods

These are better bought new, but do remember that if a domestic appliance is used in a business premises then the warranty becomes invalid.

General notes on equipment and furniture

Each piece of equipment and furniture will be expected to have a certain lifetime, electrical goods having the shortest. Take this into account in your calculations. Although you will probably pay for them as you buy them, you need to have an idea of how much they will cost you a year to write off. This will allow you to replace them in a number of years.

Computer

It is possible to manage without a computer when first starting out, although the accessibility of the Internet and the storage of useful data do make it an invaluable item.

Printers and scanners can now be bought very cheaply so adjunctive equipment may not be too expensive.

Professional fees

Membership of your professional body must be paid, and with the advent of continuing professional development some money must be set aside to fulfil this requirement.

Depending on your situation, you may have to pay for the services of an accountant and a solicitor.

Consumables

These are the small items of everyday use that are often forgotten, but are very necessary.

Sundries

These tend to consist of items for decoration and to improve the ambiance and comfort of a room and do not require great expense. You may already have many of them at home. As with all electrical appliances, new or old, get them checked so that you conform to safety legislation.

Stock

This has not been included in the examples for simplicity. Many practitioners prefer to use prescription services or have products posted on an individual basis either to patients' homes or timed to arrive before the next visit. This means that the product can be paid for by the patient in advance, not leaving the practitioner out of pocket. There is also no risk of being left with stock that has to be disposed of because it has exceeded its sell-by date.

If you do want to keep stock on the premises, work out what its shelf life is and then calculate how much it will cost you a year to keep it on your shelf:

$$\text{Cost of stock for the year} = \frac{\text{Cost of stock}}{\text{Number of years stock is viable}}$$

The result can then be added to the costings.

Analysis of pie charts calculated from fixed costs

Compare the pie charts of the costs incurred by the three therapists in the worked examples (Figs 16.1–16.3). They may appear confusing at first, but a simple analysis reveals some interesting facts.

If wages and services are added together for the chiropractor they come to 75%, in other words three-quarters, of the running cost. Most employers estimate that wages will take up a minimum of 25% of the running cost. It is worth bearing this in mind before you take on staff, as you will not easily be able to let them go without fulfilling the legal requirements of redundancy if they have been with you long enough to be entitled to this payment.

The service costs of the acupuncturist working from home are considerably smaller at 32% of running costs. Although the remedial masseur does appear to have high service charges at 63% of running cost, do not forget that he has very little in the way of equipment, and does not require to buy tables, chairs or other items necessary for equipping a clinic. The service cost also includes all the utilities and, for those who are good at negotiating, the service charge can be incurred only for the time they are working in the clinic or per patient.

Service charges are generally the one overhead you cannot adjust, because they are constant. The remedial masseur is fortunate to only incur them while at work, whereas the chiropractor, working from rented premises, and the acupuncturist largely have ongoing charges whether they are there or not.

All the other charges incurred by the remedial masseur and the acupuncturist appear quite large, and these are areas that can be adjusted to reduce costs. The chiropractor, however, because services and wages take up such a large part of the budget, may find it difficult to cut costs in the other areas, as collectively they only come to 25% of the total cost.

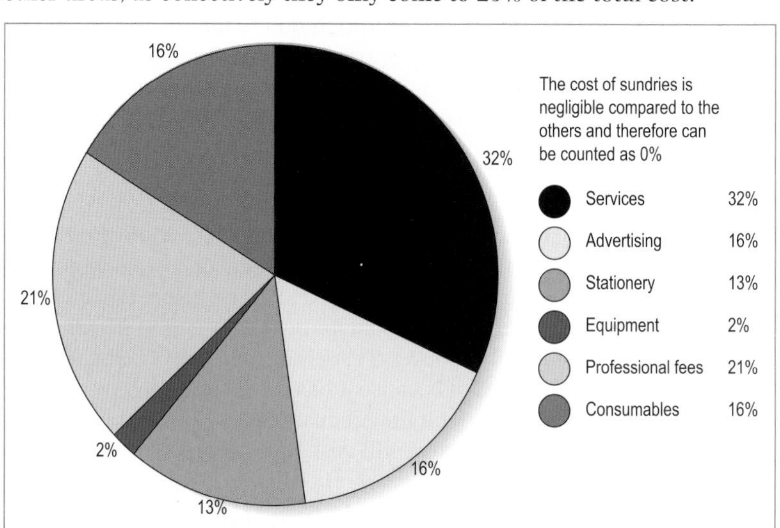

Figure 16.1 Acupuncturist: percentage breakdown of fixed costs.

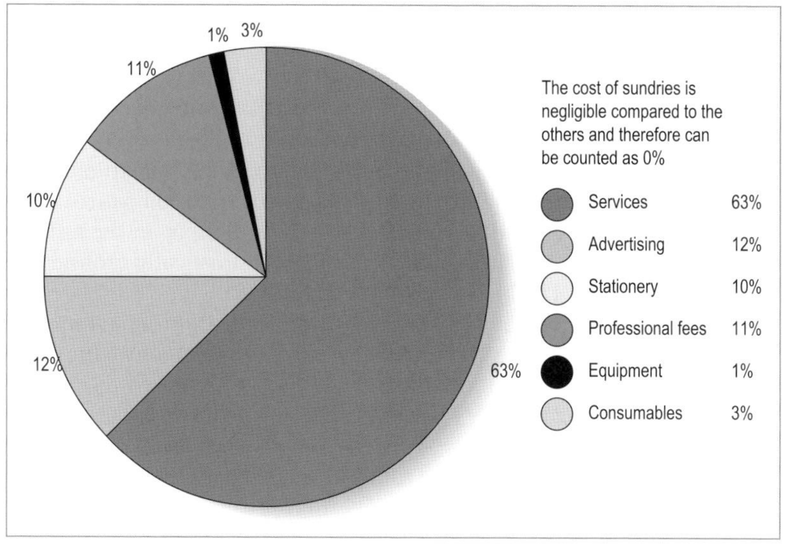

Figure 16.2 Remedial masseur: percentage breakdown of fixed costs.

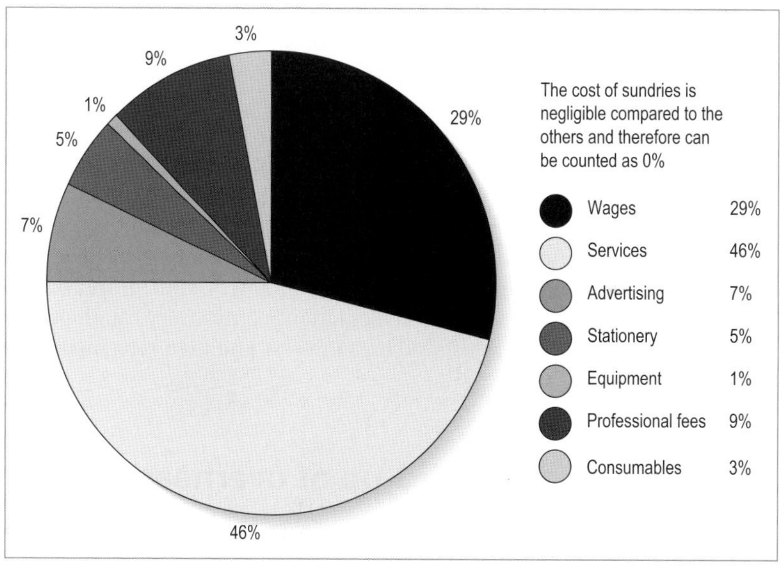

Figure 16.3 Chiropractor: percentage breakdown of fixed costs.

So how many patients a day do I have to see to break even?

The next stage is to move on to assumptions and build-up of overheads. But before you can do that it is a good idea at this stage to get a rough idea of daily running costs. The calculation to see how many patients you will need to see each day to cover the daily running costs is simple. You will, however, need to work out a price per patient to do this. So work on a basic treatment price.

The easiest way to work out your fee structure is to find out comparable charges from practitioners in your own field. Those who are very experienced or qualified in more than one area will charge higher than the average fee, but it is their special qualities that assure them of a good patient flow. These prices are the amounts that people can afford to pay in the area in which you are working. This is why fees differ so drastically around the country for the same therapy.

You may well decide that as you are less experienced you should stick to the average charge, since to charge too low a figure may not give the right impression to your potential patients.

Patients do shop around for the cheapest deal, which considering that it is their well-being that is at stake, may be a strange concept to many practitioners. Do not be tempted to take someone on as a patient for a lower fee, just because you are desperate for patients. Your professional responsibility to that patient cannot be less, purely because the patient is receiving a discounted treatment.

In all the worked examples the amount of money that would theoretically be needed in 1 year has been totalled from all the itemized lists.

The practitioners decided they would work 46 weeks a year. From this, the running cost per day of their respective clinics was calculated then divided by the treatment fee.

It is quite interesting to see that an acupuncturist working from home will require three patients a day, a remedial masseur working from a licensed room four patients a day, and a chiropractor with rented accommodation and one member of staff 10 patients a day to break even.

Once you have a price and have done the calculation, it is easy to see that increasing the size of the clinic and the addition of staff dramatically increases the running costs. But this calculation is only a very rough guide, there may possibly be other costs such as interest and loan repayments to consider.

Assumptions and build-up of overheads

Itemize everything in a logical order, although it will roughly follow your fixed cost calculations. There is no hard and fast rule, just as long as everything you can think of is noted.

By following the calculations in assumptions and build-up of overheads you will be able to break down all the items into one monthly figure for each heading, which can then be put into the cash-flow and profit/loss forecast.

Stock can probably be regarded, as far as costing out a monthly amount, in the same way as equipment without depreciation. You may at some point have to write off stock that has gone past its sell-by date, but that is irrelevant for the moment since it is too far in the future (but if you do have to write off stock, you have miscalculated and overstocked, which is an expensive mistake).

Another row for stock should be added to the cash-flow and profit/loss forecast.

The first month and last months of the years are likely to incur different charges from the rest of the months of the year. Utilities charges occur four times a year, but for simplicity's sake it has been decided to load these onto the first month and allowances have been made every third month.

Cash-flow and profit/loss forecast

The cash-flow and profit/loss forecast is your calculation as to what is going to happen over a period of time. In fact a budget. Constant reference of actual against budget will tell you how you are doing and help to act as a constant reminder to make adjustments as necessary.

Now you have calculated the cost of each general heading you will need to put them separately into the cash-flow and profit/loss forecast in each month's column. The monthly entries are then added up and the estimated living expenses added to get a total.

Only the earnings from the clinic have been included to leave a clear picture of exactly what the clinic is earning. You will be able to add income from other sources if you so wish, but the two should not be confused or you may get a false picture of how well the clinic is performing.

The income is then deducted from the total expenses to get a monthly amount.

This can look quite alarming at first, as the negative amounts can be quite large. Do not forget, however, that you are starting a new business, and unless you have sufficient savings, a certain amount of debt can be expected to be incurred, although you must be seen to be making an impression on it in the course of the year.

The deficit will initially increase then decrease and the amount become positive to show a profit. Each month is added to the previous month to be put in the cumulative column. Again, this will initially increase then decrease.

There may be monthly fluctuations in the income, which you will have estimated in the assumptions and build-up of income spreadsheets.

Assumptions and build-up of income spreadsheets

With every new business these are based on an educated guess. If you are lucky enough to know an established practitioner, see if you can get help with this. Very often someone who has established a clinic will be able to give you an idea of the speed with which business has been built up. Do try, however, to speak to a practitioner who has set up in the last 5 years, or opened a new clinic fairly recently, or your information may not be accurate.

Your market research is also a valuable asset and will also help you to make this judgement. Try to be as realistic as possible. Do not forget to include holidays; you cannot work 52 weeks of the year.

What does this all mean?

In all three scenarios in the worked examples, the practitioners have started working in their new practices full time.

In reality this is unlikely to happen unless the practitioner has a substantial amount of money saved up to afford this luxury. Many practitioners do carry on in other forms of work or working for other practitioners until they are able to build up their clinic to a point where it is self-sufficient. Working this way initially requires long working hours, fitting in patients in your own clinic at evenings or weekends or on your day off, but self-sufficiency does eventually happen and your hard work is rewarded. Meanwhile, the income from your clinic is supplemented to give you a living wage and pay off your loan or overdraft.

What does working out a budget tell you?

Spreadsheets are very easy to use and your budget can be laid out on one. The pie chart produced for each example was worked out by simply entering the annual amounts against each heading. This gives an instant picture of just how you are spending your money, which may help you to visualize the importance of each section of your budget.

By knowing roughly how much your annual spending will be, you will have a clear idea of just how big a loan you will need to ask for. You require enough money to do three things:

- *Cover living expenses.* This will include money for the occasional treat, such as a holiday or a day out, but nothing too extravagant.
- *Cover business expenses.* Allow for events such as illness and time taken off.
- *Cover the loan repayments.* Initially you are likely to be running at a loss.

Conclusion

Even if you are not applying for an overdraft or business loan, you must examine your financial situation carefully. To do so will keep you out of trouble and enable you to get out of debt much faster.

Even a rough and ready examination of the amount of money needed to get your vision going is another way of finding out the right way of initially starting your working life.

Taking the time to examine your finances properly may give you cause for a rethink at this stage. This is no bad thing, since there is nothing worse than plunging into a situation that gives you sleepless nights and anxiety.

You have now completed all the preparations necessary for your business plan.

You must have a well-thought-out budget that fits your circumstances.

You must on a regular basis, at least monthly, measure actual against budget.

Appendix 16.1

Worked example

An acupuncturist has decided to set up in a room at home.

She has consulted her accountant, as she wants to offset some of the services such as electricity and possibly the mortgage. This is a complicated part of the tax and legal system and it is important to take professional advice. If you do not you may find your home partially classed as business premises and be charged for it accordingly when you sell.

She has also had approval from the local planning office and local licensing office.

Furnishings

Assume that carpets and blinds are in place. Until the room has some history of business use it is difficult to write off such items against tax.

Services

After talking to her accountant she had decided to charge her clinic annually	£250
Acupuncture licence (one-off payment)	£50
Servicing equipment (annual)	£168
Electrical testing (annual)	£72
Telephone landline including 24/7 repair*	£500
Telephone mobile (free phone included in service)	£480
Security servicing and line monitoring (annual)†	£396
Sharps disposal (every 2 months) £18 × 6	£108
Registration of business name (annual)	£60
Data protection (annual)	£35
Business and part home insurance (annual)	£500
Services yearly	**£2619**

*24/7 repair is not absolutely necessary for priority fault repair, because the clinic phone can be transferred to your mobile or other phone at no extra cost.

†Taking security to this lengths may not be necessary but bear in mind that you will have to make your departure on holiday common knowledge.

Advertising

Yellow Pages (corporate and main)	£800
Professional leaflets (100)	£28
Local advertising	£500
Total advertising per year	**£1328**

Stationery

Printed case history forms* (100, 4 sides)	£100
Headed notepaper† (500)	£100
Business cards (200)	£80

Envelopes for letters (1000)	£10
Envelopes for case history forms (250)	£3
A4 photocopy sheets (5 reams)	£20
Sundries (paper clips, staples, stamps, etc.)	£40
Total stationery	**£353**

Assume this needs renewing every 4 months.

Stationery per year £353 × 3 **£1059**

*Case history forms do not have to be professionally printed, but can be produced on a computer and printed out on A4 sheets.
†Your headed notepaper can be used as both compliment slips and pre-printed receipts.

Equipment

Unmechanized treatment couch	£400
2 sets couch covers @ £20 each	£40
4 towels for patient covers (132 cm × 75 cm) @ £11 each	£44
2 towels for patient covers (165 cm × 100 cm) @£16	£32
1 desk	£50
1 typist chair	£25
1 patient chair	£25
Four-drawer filing cabinet (second-hand)	£50
Answering machine with cordless phone	£120
Clinic jacket	£30
Combined fax, scanner, photocopier	£200
Total	**£1016**

This is the basic list of equipment and clothing she will need to start her practice.

Now estimate the lifetime of each piece of equipment. For simplicity's sake it is a good idea to group equipment together according to the amount of time it will take to wear out. This is a generalization and equipment may have a much longer lifetime, but assume you will be replacing it.

10 Years

Treatment couch	£400
Desk	£50
Filing cabinet	£50
Total cost	**£500**
Therefore cost per year = £500/10 years =	**£50**

5 Years

1 chair	£25
1 typist chair	£25
Total cost	**£50**
Therefore cost per year = £50/5 years =	**£10**

4 Years

Couch covers	£40
Towels (132 cm × 75 cm)	£44
Towels (165 cm × 100 cm)	£32
Clinic jacket	£30
Combined printer, fax, scanner, photocopier	£200
Answering machine with cordless phone	£120
Total cost	**£466**
Therefore cost per year = £466/4 years =	**£116**

The lengths of time are an estimate and it is possible that the equipment may last much longer, but it is useful to put a time limit on it, as wear varies and you may wish to buy new equipment as time goes on.

10 years	£50
5 years	£10
4 years	£116
Total equipment cost per year	**£176**

Professional fees (yearly)

Professional membership	£600
Seminars (including accommodation)	£500
Accountant	£600
Total professional fees	**£1700**

Consumables

Head rolls	£20
Couch rolls	£18
Needles	£105
Soap	£4
Hand towels	£28
Toilet rolls	£18
Cleaning products	£15
Tea and coffee	£15
Total cost consumables	**£223**

Assume these supplies last 2 months.

Total consumables per year £223 × 6 =	**£1338**

Sundries

Pictures (framed)	£20
Plants	£10
Fans (2 @ £20)	£40
Fan heater	£30
Table lamps (2 @ £10)	£20

Floor lamps (2 @ £25)				£50
Total sundries				**£170**

Assume these last 5 years.

Total cost per year = £170/5 =	**£34**

Adding all these up to reach the total cost per year:

Services				£2619
Advertising				£1328
Stationery				£1059
Equipment				£176
Professional fees				£1700
Consumables				£1338
Sundries				£34
Total per year				**£8254**
First year	Equipment	Initial cost	£1016	
	Sundries	Initial cost	£170	£1186
Totals		**£1186**	**£9440**	

The number of working days in running the clinic for 1 year, assuming 4 days per week, 46 weeks per year = 46 × 4 = 184 working days per year

Therefore the cost per working day of running the clinic = £8254/184 = £45 per day

Cost per treatment = £25

Number of patients a day required to break even = £45/25 = 2 patients a day

If the average cost of an acupuncture treatment in the area is £25, she would need to see two patients a day to cover the running costs.

These figures are not definitive and do not include living expenses, but it is now possible to calculate how much money she would need to comfortably tide herself over until she is seeing enough patients to be financially self-sufficient.

All figures are rounded up to the nearest whole number.

Acupuncturist: assumptions and build-up of overheads

Services	£2619				
First month		**Last month**		**Basic month**	
Acupuncture licence	50	Servicing equipment	168	Total balance	£2619
Electrical test	72	Charge for room	250	Deduct	
Registration of business name	60		418	first month	1113
Data protection	35	Add basic month	82		1506
Line monitoring	396	Add sharps	18	Deduct	
Business and home insurance	500	**Total last month**	518	last month	418
	1113				1088
Add basic cost of month	82			Deduct sharps	108
Total first month	£1195				980
				Divide by 12 months =	£82 pcm
Months 2, 4, 6, 8, 10, 12					
Basic month	82				
Sharps	18				
	£100				

Months 3, 5, 7, 9, 11 are basic months	£82 pcm	
First month	1195	
2, 4, 6, 8, 10 5 months @ £100	500	
3, 5, 7, 9, 11 5 months @ £82	410	
Last month	518	
	£2623	Differential is in basic monthly calculation

Advertising **£1328**

First month		Last month	Basic month	
Yellow Pages*	800	As basic	Total for advertising	£1328
Professional leaflets	28		Deduct first month	828
	828			500
Monthly charge	42		Divide by 12 months, say	£42 pcm
First month	870		Months 1–11 =	£42 pcm
Plus 11 × £42	462			
	£1332	Differential is in monthly calculation		

*Need to find out timing of advertisement in Yellow Pages, as the publication may be part way through the financial year

Stationery	**£1059**		
Months		Total stationery renewable every 4 months	£1059
1, 5, 9	£353	£1059 divided by 3 =	£353

Equipment — **£1016 + £176 depreciation per year**
Total £1192

First month		**Monthly charge**		
Assume all equipment bought in first month		Depreciation		£176
		Divide £176 by 12 months =		
Total cost	1016	6 months @ £15	=	90
Plus monthly charge	15	6 months @ £14	=	84
	1031			174
Months				
2, 4, 6, 8, 10, 12 @ £14	84			
3, 5, 7, 9, 11 @ £15	75			
	£1190	Differential is in monthly calculation		

Professional fees — **£1700**

First month		**Monthly charge**	
Professional membership	600	Seminars	500
Accountant (part)	200	Account balance	400
Monthly charge	75		900
First month	875		
		Divided by 12 months	£75 pcm

Months 2–12 inclusive			
£75 per calendar month			
Therefore 11 × £75 =	825		
	£1700		
Consumables	**£1338**		
Months		Total consumables	£1338
1, 3, 5, 7, 9, 11 @ £223 =	£1338	Renewable every 2 months	
		£1338 divided by 6 =	£223
Sundries	**£170 + £34 depreciation per year** **Total £204**		

	First month		**Monthly charge**
	170		Depreciation £34
Monthly charge	3		Divided by 12 months, say £3 per calendar month
First month	173		
Months 2–12 @ £3	= 33		
	£206	Differential is in monthly calculation	

Acupuncturist: assumptions and build-up of income

First year

Month	Holidays (weeks)	Days worked	Patients	Rate	Total (£)
1	1	12	8	£25	200
2		16	16	£25	400
3		16	32	£25	800
4		16	48	£25	1200
5	1	12	38	£25	950
6		16	80	£25	2000
7		16	112	£25	2800
8	2	8	64	£25	1600
9	1	12	102	£25	2550
10		16	128	£25	3200
11		16	144	£25	3600
12	1	12	96	£25	2400
					21,700

Acupuncture: assumptions and build-up of income

Second year

Month	Holidays (weeks)	Days worked	Patient numbers per day	Patient numbers per month	Rate	Total (£)
1	1	12	9	108	£25	2700
2		16	9	144	£25	3600
3		16	9	144	£25	3600
4		16	9	144	£25	3600
5	1	12	9	108	£25	2700
6		16	9	144	£25	3600
7		16	9	144	£25	3600
8	2	8	9	72	£25	1800
9	1	12	9	108	£25	2700
10		16	9	144	£25	3600
11		16	9	144	£25	3600
12	1	12	9	108	£25	2700
						37,800

Acupuncturist: cash-flow and profit/loss forecast

First year

Month	1	2	3	4	5	6	7	8	9	10	11	12	
Services	1195	100	82	100	82	100	82	100	82	100	82	518	
Advertising	870	42	42	42	42	42	42	42	42	42	42	42	
Stationery	353				353				353				
Equipment	1031	14	15	14	15	14	15	14	15	14	15	14	
Professional fees	875	75	75	75	75	75	75	75	75	75	75	75	
Consumables	223		223		223		223		223		223		
Sundries	173	3	3	3	3	3	3	3	3	3	3	3	
Total	4720	234	440	234	793	234	440	234	793	234	440	652	9448
Living expenses	1666	1666	1666	1666	1666	1666	1666	1666	1666	1666	1666	1666	19,992
Total	6386	1900	2106	1900	2459	1900	2106	1900	2459	1900	2106	2318	29,440
Income	200	400	800	1200	950	2000	2800	1600	2550	3200	3600	2400	21,700
Monthly ±	–6186	–1500	–1306	–700	–1509	100	694	–300	91	1300	1494	82	
Cum ±		–7686	–8992	–9692	–11,201	–11,101	–10,407	–10,707	–10,616	–9316	–7822	–7740	c/fwd

Overdraft interest depending on amount could add £750 to £10,000 loan

Second year

Assuming overheads and living expenses (less initial cost of equipment and sundries) are as first year and income basis as per schedule

Total	5200	1900	2106	1900	2459	1900	2106	1900	2459	1900	2106	2318	28,254
Income	2700	3600	3600	3600	2700	3600	3600	1800	2700	3600	3600	2700	37,800
Monthly ±	–2500	1700	1494	1700	241	1700	1494	–100	241	1700	1494	382	
Cum b/fwd	–7740												
Cum ±	–10,240	–8540	–7046	–5346	–5105	–3405	–1911	–2011	–1770	–70	1424	1806	

Acupuncturist: revenue projections

	First year	Second year	Third year
	Overheads include purchase of equipment and £19,992 living expenses	Overheads as first year but excluding purchase of equipment	Assuming income/overheads/ living expenses remain as second year
Overheads	29,440	28,254	28,254
Income	21,700	37,800	37,800
Profit/shortfall	–7740	9546	9546
Deduct shortfall from year 1		–7740	
Net profit year 2		1806	
Net profit year 3			9546

The maximum borrowing in the first year would be £11,201

Appendix 16.2

Worked example

A remedial masseur wants to set up in a room in premises that lease rooms on a daily charge basis under licence. He has a receptionist provided in the cost to take his bookings, and use of the washroom and kitchen facilities of the clinic. All the furniture including the treatment couch is present. All services are included in the licence fee.

He is not permitted to use the clinic phone.

He intends to work a 4-day week.

He needs to work out his expenses to see what his break-even point is and how many patients a day he needs to achieve this.

Services

Licence paid monthly in advance and costs = £30 per day: £30 × 4 days × 52 weeks	£6240
Telephone mobile (free phone included in service) (monthly) £40 × 12	£480
Registration of business name (annual)	£60
Services per year including licence	**£6780**

Advertising

Yellow Pages (corporate and main)	£800
Leaflets (100)	£30
Local advertising	£500
Total advertising per year	**£1330**

Stationery

Printed case history forms* (100, 4 sides)	£100
Headed notepaper† (500)	£100
Business cards (200)	£80
Envelopes for letters (1000)	£10
Envelopes for case history forms (250)	£3
A4 photocopy sheets (5 reams)	£20
Sundries (paper clips, staples, stamps, etc.)	£40
Total stationery	**£353**

Assume this needs renewing every four months.

Stationery per year = £353 × 3 **£1059**

*Case history forms and headed notepaper do not have to be professionally printed, but can be produced on a computer and printed out on A4 sheets.

†Your headed notepaper can be used as both compliment slips and pre-printed receipts.

Professional fees (yearly)

Professional membership	£130
Seminars (including accommodation)	£500
Accountant	£600
Total professional fees per year	**£1230**

Equipment

Four-drawer filing cabinet (second-hand)	£50
Answering machine with cordless phone	£120
Clinic jacket	£30
Combined fax, photocopier	£200
Couch covers 2 @ £20	£40
Towels 6 @ £10	£60
Total	**£500**

Now estimate the lifetime of each piece of equipment. For simplicity's sake it is a good idea to group the equipment together according to the amount of time it will take to wear out. This is a generalization, and equipment may have a much longer lifetime, but assume you will be replacing it.

10 Years

Four-drawer filing cabinet will last at least 10 years

Therefore per year the cabinet costs £50/10 =	**£5**

4 Years

Clinic jacket	£30
Couch covers	£40
Towels	£60
Combined fax, photocopier	£200
Answering machine with cordless phone	£120
Total cost	**£450**
Therefore cost per year = £450/4 years =	**£113**

The lengths of time are an estimate and it is possible that the equipment may last much longer, but it is useful to put a time limit on it, as wear varies and you may wish to buy new equipment as time goes on.

10 years	£5
4 years	£113
Total equipment cost per year	**£118**

Consumables

Massage cream	£30
Couch rolls	£18
Total	**£48**

Assume these supplies last 2 months.

Total consumables over 1 year = £48 × 6 = £288

Adding all these up to reach the total cost per year:

Services	£6780
Advertising	£1330
Stationery	£1059
Professional fees	£1230
Equipment	£118
Consumables	£288

Total per year		**£10,805**
First year	Equipment initial cost	£500
Total		**£11,305**

The number of working days in running the clinic, assuming 4 days per week, 46 weeks per year = 46 × 4 = 184 working days per year

Therefore the cost per working day of running the clinic = £11,305/184 = £62 per day

Cost per treatment = £33

Number of patients a day required to break even = £62/33 = 2 patients a day

If the average cost of a massage treatment in the area is £33, he would need to see two patients a day to cover the running costs.

These figures are not definitive and do not include living expenses, but it is now possible to calculate how much money he would need to borrow to comfortably tide him over until he is seeing enough patients to be financially self-sufficient.

All figures are rounded up to the nearest whole number.

Remedial masseur: assumptions and build-up of overheads

Services **£6780**

First month			Basic month		
Registration of business name	60		Total service		£6780
	60		Deduct		
Add basic cost for month	560		first month		60
Total first month	620				6720
First month	620		Divide by 12 months	=	£560 pcm
Months 2–12 = 11 × £560	6160				
	£6780				

Advertising **£1330**

First month		Last month	Basic month	
Yellow Pages*	800	Deduct	Total for advertising	£1330

Professional leaflets	30	as basic	Deduct first month	830
	830			500
Monthly charge	42		Divide by 12 months, say	£42 pcm
First month	870		Months 1–12 =	£42 pcm
Plus months 2–12 = 11 @ £42	462			
	£1332	Differential is in monthly calculation		

*Need to find out timing of advertisement in Yellow Pages, as the publication may be part way through the financial year

Stationery	**£1059**			
			Total stationery renewable every 4 months	£1059
Months				
1, 5, 9 @ £353 =	£1059		Therefore £1059 divided by 3 = £353	

Equipment **£500 + £118 depreciation each year**
Total £618

First month			Monthly charge	
Assume all equipment bought in first month			Depreciation	£118
Total cost	500		Divided by 12 months, say	
Plus monthly charge	9		6 months @ £10	60
First month	509		6 months @ £9	54
				114
Months				
2, 4, 6, 8, 10, 12 @ £10 pcm	60			
3, 5, 7, 9, 11 @ £9 pcm	45			
	£614	Differential is in monthly calculation		

Professional fees	**£1230**		
First month		**Monthly charge**	
Professional membership	130	Seminars	500
Accountant (part)	200	Accountant balance	400
	330		900

Monthly charge	75		
First month	405	Divided by 12 months =	£75 pcm
Months 2–12 inclusive =			
11 months @ £75	825		
	£1230		
Consumables	**£288**		
		Total consumables	£288
		Renewable every 2 months	
Months 1, 3, 5, 7, 9, 11 @ £48 =	£288	Therefore £288 divided by 6 =	£48
		every 2 calendar months	
Sundries	**Nil**		

Remedial masseur: assumptions and build-up of income

First year

Month	Holidays (weeks)	Days worked	Patients	Rate	Total (£)
1	1	12	7	£33	231
2		16	12	£33	396
3		16	18	£33	594
4		16	25	£33	825
5	1	12	17	£33	561
6		16	28	£33	924
7		16	32	£33	1056
8	2	8	18	£33	594
9	1	12	36	£33	1188
10		16	64	£33	2112
11		16	80	£33	2640
12	1	12	60	£33	1980
					13,101

Remedial masseur: assumptions and build-up of income

Second year

Month	Holidays (weeks)	Days worked	Patient numbers per day	Patient numbers per month	Rate	Total (£)
1	1	12	7	84	£33	2772
2		16	7	112	£33	3696
3		16	7	112	£33	3696
4		16	7	112	£33	3696
5	1	12	7	84	£33	2772
6		16	7	112	£33	3696
7		16	7	112	£33	3696
8	2	8	7	56	£33	1848
9	1	12	7	84	£33	2772
10		16	7	112	£33	3696
11		16	7	112	£33	3696
12	1	12	7	84	£33	2772
						38,808

Remedial masseur: cash-flow and profit/loss forecast

First year

Month	1	2	3	4	5	6	7	8	9	10	11	12	
Services	620	560	560	560	560	560	560	560	560	560	560	560	
Advertising	870	42	42	42	42	42	42	42	42	42	42	42	
Stationery	353				353				353				
Equipment	509	10	9	10	9	10	9	10	9	10	9	10	
Professional fees	405	75	75	75	75	75	75	75	75	75	75	75	
Consumables	48		48		48		48		48		48		
Sundries	N/A	N/A	N/A	N/A	N/A	N/A	N/A	N/A	N/A	N/A	N/A	N/A	
Total	2805	687	734	687	1087	687	734	687	1087	687	734	687	11,303
Living expenses	1250	1250	1250	1250	1250	1250	1250	1250	1250	1250	1250	1250	15,000
Total	4055	1937	1984	1937	2337	1937	1984	1937	2337	1937	1984	1937	26,303
Earnings (Incl. other clinic)	231	396	594	825	561	924	1056	594	1188	2112	2640	1980	13,101
Monthly ±	–3824	–1541	–1390	–1112	–1776	–1013	–928	–1343	–1149	175	656	43	
Cum ±		–5365	–6755	–7867	–9643	–10,656	–11,584	–12,972	–14,076	–13,901	–13,245	–13,202	c/fwd

Overdraft interest depending on amount could add £750 to £10,000 loan

Second year

Assuming overheads and living expenses (less initial cost of equipment) are as first year and income basis as per schedule

Total	3555	1937	1984	1937	2337	1937	1984	1937	2337	1937	1984	1937	25,803
Income	2772	3696	3696	3696	2772	3696	3696	1848	2772	3696	3696	2772	38,808
Monthly ±	–783	1759	1712	1759	435	1759	1712	–89	435	1759	1712	835	
Cum b/fwd	–13,202												
Cum ±	–13,985	–12,226	–10,514	–8755	–8320	–6561	–4849	–4938	–4503	–2744	–1032	–197	

Remedial masseur: revenue projections

	First year	**Second year**	**Third year**
	Overhead include purchase of equipment and £15,000 living expenses	Overheads as first year but excluding purchase of equipment	Assuming income/overheads/ living expenses remain as second year
Overheads	26,303	25,803	25,803
Income	13,101	38,808	38,808
Profit/shortfall	–13,202	13,005	13,005
Deduct shortfall from year 1		13,202	
Net loss year 2		–197	
Deduct loss for second year			–197
Net profit year 3			12,808

The maximum borrowing in the first year would be £14,076

Appendix 16.3

Worked example

A chiropractor wants to set up in rented premises, which consist of two main rooms, a small kitchen area and toilet facilities. One room will be a reception with a receptionist, the other room a treatment room.

She needs to work out her expenses to see what her break-even point is.

Furnishings

Assume that carpets and blinds are supplied.

Wages for a receptionist (including PAYE and National Insurance)

Assume £8 per hour, 8 hours per day, 4 days per week, 52 weeks per year.
8 hours per day × 4 days per weeks = 32 hours per week.
32 hours per week × 52 weeks per year = 1664 hours per year

1664 hours per year × £8 =	**£13,312**

Services per year (based on a 4-week month)

Rent 50 square metres (538 square feet): assume £18 per square foot per year	£9684
Water (quarterly) £114 × 4	£456
Electricity (quarterly) £75 × 4	£300
Gas (quarterly) £75 × 4	£300
Insurance for boiler breakdown (annual)	£180
Window cleaner (monthly) £15 × 12	£180
Cleaning premises (weekly) £32 × 52	£1664
Servicing equipment (annual)	£168
Electrical testing (annual)	£72
Telephone landline including 24/7 repair	£800
Telephone mobile (free phone included in service) (monthly) £40 × 12	£480
Broadband (monthly) £20 × 12	£240
Security servicing and line monitoring (annual)	£396
Sharps disposal (every 3 months) £12 × 4	£48
Local council rates (monthly) £83 × 12	£996
Refuse collection (monthly) £35 × 12	£420
Registration of business name (annual)	£60
Data protection (annual)	£35
Vehicle hire purchase (monthly) £220 × 12	£2640
Business insurance (annual)	£900
Vehicle insurance (annual)	£400
Road fund licence (annual)	£120
Vehicle servicing and parts (annual)	£400

Wages and services annually	**£34,251**

It is the responsibility of the owner of the building to ensure legislation regarding fire safety is complied with, so costs for this are not included.

Advertising

Yellow Pages (corporate and main)	£1300
Professional leaflets (300)	£90
Local advertising	£2000
Total advertising per year	**£3390**

Stationery

Printed treatment record sheets* (100, 4 sides)	£100
Headed notepaper* (500)	£100
Business cards (200)	£80
Envelopes for letters (1000)	£10
Envelopes for treatment record sheets (250)	£3
Compliment slips† (500)	£100
Pre-printed receipts† (500)	£100
A4 photocopy sheets (5 reams)	£20
Sundries (paper clips, staples, stamps, etc.)	£40
Total stationery	**£533**

Assume this needs renewing every 3 months.

Total stationery per year = £533 × 4	**£2132**

*Treatment record sheets and headed notepaper do not have to be professionally printed, but can be produced on a computer and printed out on A4 sheets.
†Your headed notepaper can be used as both compliment slips and pre-printed receipts.

Equipment

Treatment couch (new, portable with drops)	£1000
4 Sets couch covers @ £10 each	£40
15 Patient gowns @ £15 each	£225
2 Desks @ £50 each	£100
2 Typist chairs @ £25 each	£50
4 Reception chairs @ £25 each	£100
Four-drawer filing cabinet (second-hand)	£50
Answering machine with cordless phone	£120
Clinic jacket	£30
Computer	£900
Combined fax, scanner, photocopier	£200
Vacuum cleaner	£70
Table-top fridge	£110
Microwave	£70
Total	**£3065**

This is the basic list of equipment and clothing she will need to start her practice.

The figures include all the connection cables required, monitor, speakers, CPU, mouse, CD re-writer, etc. and office software, from a specialist firm.

Bear in mind that the warranty for any electrical equipment will be void if it is for business use. You will have to contact the individual retailers for information on this.

Now estimate the lifetime of each piece of equipment. For simplicity's sake it is a good idea to group the equipment together according to the amount of time it will take to wear out. This is a generalization and equipment may have a much longer lifetime, but assume you will be replacing it.

10 Years

Treatment couch	£1000
2 desks	£100
Filing cabinet	£50
Total cost	**£1150**
Therefore cost per year = £1150/10 years =	**£115**

5 Years

Vacuum	£70
Fridge	£110
Microwave	£70
4 chairs	£100
2 typist chairs	£50
Total cost	**£400**
Therefore cost per year = £400/5 years =	**£80**

4 Years

Clinic jacket	£30
Couch covers	£40
Patient gowns	£225
Computer	£900
Combined printer, fax, scanner	£200
Answering machine with cordless phone	£120
Total cost	**£1515**
Therefore cost per year = £1515/4 years =	**£379**

The lengths of time are an estimate and it is possible that the equipment may last much longer, but it useful to put a time limit on it, as wear varies and you may wish to buy new equipment as time goes on.

10 years	£115
5 years	£80
4 years	£379

Total equipment cost per year **£574**

Professional fees (yearly)

Register membership	£1000
Professional membership	£900
Seminars (including accommodation)	£2000
Accountant	£600
Solicitor (reading rental agreement and drawing up contract)	£400

Total professional fees per year **£4900**

Consumables

Head rolls	£20
Couch rolls	£18
Needles	£105
Soap	£4
Hand towels	£28
Toilet rolls	£18
Cleaning products	£15
Tea and coffee	£15

Total **£223**

Assume these supplies last 2 months.

Total consumables over 1 year = 223 × 6 = **£1338**

Sundries

Pictures (framed)	£20
Plants	£10
Fans (2 @ £20)	£40
Fan heater	£30
Table lamps (2 @ £10)	£20
Floor lamps (2 @ £25)	£50

Total sundries **£170**

Assume these last 5 years.

Total cost per year = £170/5 = **£34**

Adding all these up to reach the total cost per year:

Services	£34,251
Advertising	£3390
Stationery	£2132
Equipment	£574
Professional fees	£4900

Consumables				£1338
Sundries				£34
Total per year				**£46,619**
First year	Equipment	Initial cost	£3065	
	Sundries	Initial cost	£170	£3235
Totals			**£3235**	**£49,854**

The number of working days in running the clinic for 1 year, assuming 4 days per week, 46 weeks per year = 46 × 4 = 184 working days per year

Therefore the cost per working day of running the clinic = £46,619/184 = £253 per day

Cost per treatment = £25

Number of patients a day required to break even = £253/25 = 10 patients a day

If the average cost of a chiropractic treatment in the area is £25, she would need to see 10 patients a working day to cover the running costs.

These figures are not definitive and do not include living expenses, but it is now possible to see how much money she would need to comfortably tide her over until she is seeing enough patients to be financially self-sufficient.

All figures are rounded up to the nearest whole number.

Chiropractor: assumptions and build-up of overheads

Services	**£34,251**			
First month		**Last month**		
Insurance for boiler	180	Servicing equipment	168	
Electrical testing	72	Basic month cost	2568	
Registration of business name	60		2736	
Data protection	35	Basic third month	276	
Line monitoring	396	Total last month	3012	
Business insurance	900			
Vehicle insurance	400			
Road fund licence	120			
	2163	**Basic month**		
Add basic cost of month	2568	Wages plus		
Total first month	4731	service		£34,251
		Deduct		
		First month	2163	
		Last month	168	
		Sharps	48	
		Water	456	

Electricity	300	
Gas	300	
	3435	3435
		30,816

Every third month				
Basic month cost		2568		
Sharps	48			
Water	456			
Gas	300		Divide by 12 months	£2568 pcm
Electricity	300			
	1104			
Divided by 4 =		276		
		2844 pcm		

First month		**4731**
Months 2, 4, 5, 7, 8, 10, 11 =	7 × 2568	17,976
Months 3, 6, 9 =	3 × 2844	8532
Last month		3012
		£34,251

Advertising **£3390**

First month			Basic month	
Yellow Pages*	1300		Total for advertising	3390
Professional leaflets	90		Deduct first month	1390
	1390			2000
Monthly charge	167			
	1557		Divided by 12 months, say	167
			2–12 @ £167	
Months				
2–12 = 11 @ £167	1837			
	£3394	Differential is in monthly calculation		

*Need to find out timing of advertisement in Yellow Pages, as the publication may be part way through the financial year

Stationery **£2132**

		Total stationery	£2132
		Renewable every 3 months	
		Therefore divide by 4	£533
Months 1, 4, 7, 10 =	£533		
4 × 533 =	£2132		

Equipment **£3065 initial cost + £574 depreciation per year**
Total £3639

First month			Monthly charge	
Assume all equipment bought in first month			Depreciation	£574
Total cost plus depreciation	3065		Divided by 12 months, say	£48 pcm
	48			
	3113			
Months				
2–12 = 11 × 48	528			
	£3641	Differential is in monthly calculation		

Professional fees **£4900**

First month		Monthly charge	
Register membership	1000	Seminars	2000
Professional membership	900	Accountant balance	400
Accountant (part)	200		2400
Solicitor	400		
Monthly charge	200	Divided by 12 months =	£200 pcm
	2700		

Months 2–12 = 11 × £200	2200		
	£4900		

Consumables	**£1338**		
Months			
1, 3, 5, 7, 9, 11		Total consumables	£1338
6 × £223 =	£1338	Renewable every 2 months	
		Therefore £1338 divided	
		by 6 = £223	

Sundries	**£170 + £34 depreciation per year**	
First month	**Total £204**	
Assume all sundries bought in first month Months 2–12 @ £3 pcm		Depreciation £34
Monthly charge	170	Divided by 12 months, say £3 pcm
	3	
First month	173	
Months 2–12 = 11 × £3 pcm	33	
	£206	Differential is in monthly calculation

Chiropractor: assumptions and build-up of income

First year

Month	Holidays (weeks)	Days worked	Patients		Patients		Amount (£)	Total (£)
			New	Rate	Repeat	Rate		
1	1	12	4	£50			200	
					12	£25	300	500
2		16	16	£50			800	
					40	£25	1000	1800
3		16	18	£50			900	
					112	£25	2800	3700
4		16	20	£50			1000	
					128	£25	3200	4200
5	1	12	16	£50			800	
					108	£25	2700	3500
6		16	22	£50			1100	
					160	£25	4000	5100
7		16	24	£50			1200	
					176	£25	4400	5600
8	2	8	13	£50			650	
					96	£25	2400	3050
9	1	12	21	£50			1050	
					156	£25	3900	4950
10		16	30	£50			1500	
					224	£25	5600	7100
11		16	32	£50			1600	
					240	£25	6000	7600
12	1	12	21	£50			1050	
					180	£25	4500	5550
								52,650

Chiropractor: assumptions and build-up of income

Second year

Income per month based on the following – 3 new patients per day + 18 repeat patients per day

16 days × 3 = 58 patients × £50 = £2900
16 days × 18 = 288 patients × £25 = £7200
Therefore 16-day month = £10,100

8 days × 3 = 24 patients × £50 = £1200
8 days × 18 = 144 patients × £25 = £3600
Therefore 8-day month = £4800

12 days × 3 = 36 patients × £50 = £1800
12 days × 18 = 216 patients × £25 = £5400
Therefore 12-day month = £7200

Month	Holidays (weeks)	Days worked	Income per month
1	1	12	7200
2		16	10,100
3		16	10,100
4		16	10,100
5	1	12	7200
6		16	10,100
7		16	10,100
8	2	8	4800
9	1	12	7200
10		16	10,100
11		16	10,100
12	1	12	7200
			104,300

Chiropractor: cash-flow and profit/loss forecast

First year

Month	1	2	3	4	5	6	7	8	9	10	11	12	
Services	4731	2568	2844	2568	2568	2844	2568	2568	2844	2568	2568	3012	
Advertising	1557	167	167	167	167	167	167	167	167	167	167	167	
Stationery	533			533			533			533			
Equipment	3113	48	48	48	48	48	48	48	48	48	48	48	
Professional fees	2700	200	200	200	200	200	200	200	200	200	200	200	
Consumables	223		223		223		223		223		223		
Sundries	173	3	3	3	3	3	3	3	3	3	3	3	
Total	13,030	2986	3485	3519	3209	3262	3742	2986	3485	3519	3209	3430	49,862
Living expenses	2400	2400	2400	2400	2400	2400	2400	2400	2400	2400	2400	2400	28,800
Total	15,430	5386	5885	5919	5609	5662	6142	5386	5885	5919	5609	5830	
Income (Incl. other clinic)	500	1800	3700	4200	3500	5100	5600	3050	4950	7100	7600	5550	52,650
Monthly ±	–14,930	–3586	–2185	–1719	–2109	–562	–542	–2336	–935	1181	1991	–280	
Cum ±		–18,516	–20,701	–22,420	–24,529	–25,091	–25,633	–27,969	–28,904	–27,723	–25,732	–26,012	c/fwd

Overdraft interest depending on amount could add £2000 to £26,268 loan

Second year

Assuming overheads and living expenses (less initial cost of equipment and sundries) are as first year, and income basis as per monthly schedule

Total	12,183	5386	5885	5919	5609	5662	6142	5386	5885	5919	5609	5830	75,415
Income	7200	10,100	10,100	10,100	7200	10,100	10,100	4800	7200	10,100	10,100	7200	104,300
Monthly ±	–4983	4714	4215	4181	1591	4438	3958	–586	1315	4181	4491	1370	
Cum b/fwd	–26,012												
Cum ±	30,995	–26,281	–22,066	–17,885	–16,294	–11,856	–7898	–8484	–7169	–2988	1503	2873	

Chiropractor: revenue projections

	First year	Second year	Third year
	Overheads include purchase of equipment and £28,800 living expenses	Overheads as first year but excluding purchase of equipment	Assuming income/overheads/ living expenses remain as second year
Overheads	78,662	75,415	75,415
Income	52,650	104,300	104,300
Profit/shortfall	–26,012	28,885	28,885
Deduct shortfall from year 1		–26,012	
Net profit year 2		2873	
Net profit year 3			28,885

The maximum borrowing in the first year would be £28,904

Putting a business plan together

17

Chapter contents

Consider a business plan in the same way you would the treatment of a patient. You do not treat a patient without first taking a proper case history, performing an examination and making an assessment of your findings. Many new practitioners regard a business plan as an unnecessary hurdle placed in their way, when in fact it is a vital document, which can help to guide them in their first few years.

The business plan is the culmination of all your previous research. This is where you bring together your market research, formulate ideas for advertising and promotion and summarize all your financial considerations.

Most banks have a ready-made business plan that requires you to fill in the appropriate spaces. This is designed with a conventional business in mind where selling products is the key means of earning money, or the owners will have several members of staff to help them run the business. Your needs may be very much simpler than this, but it is still possible to fill out most of the points in the form.

The bank business plan never leaves much space to fill out details, but the limited space clearly indicates the need for being concise. Though it appears to be relatively simple to complete, you will only be able to do so if you have the relevant amount of information to hand.

Should you decide to prepare your own business plan, the bank business plan does provide a useful format from which to prepare your own business plan.

Why is preparing your own business plan necessary?

Preparing your own business plan from scratch is very time consuming. It may not be necessary in every case, as practitioners may be setting up modestly enough not to need a loan. Producing your own business plan, however, may be one of the most valuable learning experiences of your business life, since it will make you very aware of the financial demands your business is likely to make on you and the professionalism you will require to secure a loan.

It is a vital document for both your lender and yourself, to make sure you have thought through the setting up and running of your business. A business plan gives you a clear picture of what you are about and what you want to achieve. In other words, you have a road map of where your business will be going and how it is going to get there. If your business plan does not make sense, then your business is likely to run into trouble very quickly.

It provides you with a map, which will give you a better understanding of what your business is all about and whether your ideas are financially viable. It will also provide a convincing outline to any organization you approach with a view to raising finance.

How do I start to write a business plan?

Keep the language plain and simple. It is all too easy, having spent a considerable amount of time in study, to forget that the rest of the world does not share your in-depth knowledge. Certain technical terms you are familiar with may not be understood.

You will be one of many people attempting to get a small business loan. Those who are successful will have been able to convince their lenders that they will remain viable because they have produced a business plan that is realistic and is a workable tool they can refer to, enabling them to stay viable. You have to persuade the lenders that you are one of these people. Your planning will need to carry you through the initial phase of opening a business to the next stage of growth.

Always make allowances for financial emergencies. Many small businesses get into trouble very quickly because they have not allowed themselves a generous enough financial margin to help them over the problems that may occur. These might be such things as a slower than expected build-up in patient load, a competitor opening up close by, or an economic factor such as a mortgage rate rise, which will affect not only your patients, but you as well.

A business plan that is well thought out and carefully put together will demonstrate your commitment to your business, your professionalism and the high standards you work to.

A well-prepared business plan is useless without a confident presentation. Many lenders may have had no previous exposure to complementary medicine. Be very sure you can be succinct about what it is you do and present it in a way they can relate to, by avoiding technical jargon and complex explanations. The simplest way is to describe what you can treat and expand as required from there. Your confidence in your chosen profession will be a very large part of how well the business plan can be appreciated.

In the appendix to this chapter is an example of a business plan based on the chiropractor in Appendix 16.3, who set up in rented accommodation with one member of staff. All the points in the discussion below are numbered to relate them to their counterparts in the example business plan so that it is easier to cross-reference.

The structure of the business plan

Cover page

The cover page should say the words 'Business Plan'. *(1)*

You should include.

- *Name and business name. (2)* Your name and the business you are trading under. If you wish to protect this name you can register it with the National Business Register plc. This can be done online (see p. 220) or by mail.
- *Company logo. (3)* This is not absolutely necessary, but is a nice touch. There are many copyright-free symbols available, or design your own. It may be possible to get one professionally designed for you at relatively little expense. A good logo is important, as this will be the public image you wish to project.
- *Address. (4)* Probably your home address if you do not currently have premises.
- *Telephone number. (5)* Both address and telephone number are vital if you want to be contacted. Make sure the telephone number you give has an answering machine if no one is permanently available to take messages. It is perfectly acceptable to give your mobile phone number.
- *Fax number.* If you have one.
- *Email address. (6)* This is used more commonly these days and is a quick way of communicating.
- *Date. (7)* Do not forget to put this on.

Executive summary

This is a summary of the whole business plan. Because it is likely to be the part of the document that is read first, it is crucial to get it right. It is therefore important to consider that the executive summary could be read as a stand-alone document.

It should be:

- Clear.
- Logical.
- Interesting.
- Exciting.

Opinions vary as to whether you should write the executive summary first or after the rest of the business plan. Whichever way you do it, you will need to put down key points in a logical order.

Like a good book, you are trying to grip the reader. By the time your readers have finished the executive summary they should feel enthusiastic about what you offer, and be eager to read through the rest of the document. Your readers will also have a grasp of what it is you do and what they can expect from the rest of the plan.

The impact of the executive summary should reflect in the whole document.

The summary should be no more than two to three pages long. If it ambles on it will no longer appear professional and concise. This makes it, probably, the most difficult part of the document to write.

By the time you have finished writing the executive summary you should have achieved the following:

- *Being clear in your own mind what you are trying to achieve.* The summary will force you to encapsulate what you are trying to do in setting up a clinic and where you see it going.
- *Prioritizing.* Both the business plan and the summary have a logical order to them. Because you have to be succinct you will pick out the salient points that are the most important to the success of your business.
- *An ability to write about the business more easily.* You will have headings and key ideas you can enlarge on or justify.

There are several factors you need to think through:

- *Business concept.* What market will your therapy serve? What is its competitive advantage?
- *Who are the key personnel in your clinic?* Unless you have set up in partnership, this will be you as owner and practitioner. If you have a member of staff in mind, for example a receptionist who is very experienced and has an in-depth knowledge of the complementary field, then this is worth mentioning. The receptionist's input to your clinic may be a key factor in its success.
- *What market research have you done to show that the business is viable?* You do not need to go into detail in the executive summary, just use it as a taster to draw the reader in.

- *What have you achieved so far?* You have qualified in your particular therapy. This is a very important piece of information, particularly as some courses can last up to 4 years or more. Study over this length of time or at a college recognized by a professional body shows commitment.

  Membership of a recognized body can also be an important factor in the lender's decision to give you a loan.
- *Financial features.* How do you expect to build? What do you expect to be able to bring in over what period of time? Answers to these questions show that you have thought through the rate at which your business is going to grow.
- *Financial requirements.* Do you have any assets you can use? Do you need a 100% loan?

The summary should describe the following:

- *The stage you are at in respect to your start-up. (8)* Have you already been seeing patients, or do you have premises in mind that you want to work from?
- *If it is already up and running, the people who are working at the clinic.* This might be you and a partner or a friend helping with the administration.
- *The therapy you are using to treat patients. (9)*
- *The location of the clinic. (10)*
- *A brief personal résumé. (11)*
- *The reasons why patients will come to see you. (12)*
- *Indication of market size and growth. (13)*
- *A brief résumé of your marketing strategy. (14)*
- *A summary of forecasts, income, profits and cash flow. (15)*
- *How much money you will need. (16)* For this you need to look at the cumulative (Cum ±) rows of the cash-flow and profit/loss forecast.

Have someone read your executive summary and give you an opinion. You will be unique if you do not have to re-write it several times.

Table of contents *(17)*

This is important, since it gives the reader a quick and easy way of finding each section.

All the pages of your business plan should be numbered. Once you have completed your plan, go back to the table of contents and insert the page numbers. List not only the main headings, but also subsections.

The industry

This will describe the particular therapy you use. This *may* include facts such as:

- *Numbers of people suffering from conditions that would benefit from your treatment.* These are usually easily accessed from various statistics. *(18)*

- *How long your treatment has been around. (19)* A well-established therapy may be seen as favourable. A new therapy, however, that appears to have good growth, may appear to be a good investment. Show the lender how you know this. This may be from information in a newspaper or magazine article or from your own professional body. Do make a note of your sources.
- *How many therapists there are in the country. (20)*
- *Your professional body and what it means to belong to it. (21)*
- *What may happen in the future. (22)* Are there likely to be any restrictions on practice? Will legislation improve the public perception of your therapy?
- *If there is growth in the profession, why it is happening. (23)* A simple statement of how much the market is likely to grow is not enough, and a reason why growth is occurring needs to be given. For example, an acupuncturist may be able to say that stress in the workplace is on the increase and that acupuncture has been shown to help. The acupuncturist will then quote the sources of the statement.
- *Whether any well-known people use the treatment, or any other relevant newsworthy item.* Celebrity use of a therapy is always of interest as it raises public awareness. Or substantial research projects that have been recently conducted may lead to increased use of your therapy. *(24)*

It is important to back up your statements with factual information, so that they do not appear to be conjecture designed to impress. As well as referring to professional journals, newspapers and magazines, consult your professional organization, which may well have useful statistics to hand.

If there is anything negative concerning your therapy, discuss the problems your business may face and turn it to your advantage. For example, adverse reactions to Chinese herbs reported in the press are as a result of the profession being unregulated, but the professional body you belong to is working towards the type of registration that has benefited the chiropractic and osteopathic professions. This shows you have a realistic view of the market.

Business description

You must be able to present a clear description of your business, which includes:

- *The name of the business. (25)* The lender will be expecting the name to reflect the type of business you are conducting. Check with the business names register that the name you have chosen is not being used. If it is not, then register it. There is a very reasonable fee.
  - *National Business Register plc.* Their website (see p. 220) enables you to check for business names and register your business as a sole trader, company, etc. You can also check and register your domain name and register trademarks.

- *Companies House.* This is where you will register your company name (see p. 219).
- *Nominet.* This is the UK site for checking and registering UK domain names (see p. 220).

- *The service you are offering. (26)* This is the therapy or therapies you practice.
- *Location of business.* Enlarge on the exact location of the premises, as this will have a bearing on how sensible you have been with choice of location. Also describe the topography of the building you are in, so that the lender has a picture of how much area is involved and the facilities available to you for the money you will be spending. *(27)*
- *The market that you will be accessing.* Local area, age groups, etc. Appropriately referenced statistics are important. *(28)*
- *Why your business idea is viable. (29)*

The descriptions only need to be brief as they will be covered or justified in more detail later.

What are your plans for your business (Objectives)? *(30)*

This is something you have already considered but the business plan will force you to define it more precisely.

The lender will expect you to set long-term and short-term goals, not only financially but also for your business. You may also have to list a set of achievements over a period of up to 3 years or more. This time frame is crucial, as this is the period in which many businesses suddenly find they have financial problems.

- *Your short-term financial goal* may be breaking even over the next 2 years. This consideration must take into account personal expenses. Many people starting a business forget that they also have to live.
- *Your short-term business goal* may be building up a patient load to a certain percentage of your total capacity.
- *Your long-term financial goal* may be generating enough money to buy your own premises.
- *Your long-term business goal* may be establishing a multipractitioner clinic.

These factors combined with what you want to achieve over the next few years will show you have a clear direction in which you want to take your business. Your goals or achievements do not have to be ambitious, but show lenders that your intention is to use their money wisely and prosper.

Your language should be concise and in plain English. People who ramble and use incomprehensible technical terms, for example treating 'biomechanical spinal conditions' when they could just say 'bad backs and necks', are perceived as having no business vision. If you are able to present your business plan clearly, then you will be seen as someone who understands her business and you will avoid alienating the reader.

Your clinic

Mission statement *(31)*

You should have already defined this before performing your market research (see Ch. 10).

Describing your clinic

This enables you to discuss your business in more detail. This, like the executive summary, is like a story, so while giving the facts it should be made to be as interesting as possible.

- *What type of therapy is it (nature of company)?* Although this has already been stated, it is necessary to reiterate exactly what sort of therapy you do. For example, herbal treatment with nutritional considerations. *(32)*
- *When are you intending to open the clinic?* This gives a timescale for your lenders. *(33)*
- *What type of business is it (ownership and management)?* Is there a sole proprietor or is it a partnership? *(34)*
- *Who is the principal of the clinic and what experience does she have (ownership and management)?* This will be you if you are the sole proprietor and your experience will be the training you have done. If you have a relevant biomedical qualification, for example you were a physiotherapist or biochemist, mention it. If clinical training was part of your course, then mention it and where you qualified. Your professional membership is also worth citing. *(34)*
- *Do you have any staff and what do they bring to the clinic?* Your staff may have had previous receptionist experience and strong local connections, which will help to promote your clinic. *(35)*

Description of the services you provide

Although certain therapies are self-evident, for example a herbalist will use herbs, it is still necessary to describe the conditions that can be treated and the type of management skills the therapist gives people to encourage well-being.

Stress your unique selling point (USP). *(36)* This is what sets you apart from your competitors. It is important to have some way to differentiate yourself and it is based on the features of your service.

It may be that you have spotted a niche in the market for treating a condition about which very little is being done, or a new way of managing it. For example, an aromatherapist who is an active member of a mother and toddler group has spotted a niche in the market for treatment of babies with colic and decides to deliver a treatment package for both the baby and the stressed parents, in conjunction with management techniques for the parents. This may be something no one else in the area has considered doing and is the type of USP the lenders will be looking for.

Although you will have trained to treat all conditions, investigate areas that have not yet been fully developed. This may be an opportunity, while still studying, to explore a particular area for a thesis. The thesis and the fact that it is your research will make you an expert in that particular area and is likely to impress your lender.

If your USP is successful then you are likely to have imitators. How are you going to stay ahead of the competition? Be very specific about what gives you your intended competitive edge. *(37)*

The market

This is where you will have to convince your lender that your therapy is part of a growing market. You may well have included some statistics in your section on your industry and business description. *(18, 28)* Statistics are useful, as they will provide solid evidence to back up your statements. This will prove to your lender that you have understood your market.

Introduction

You have already included some information about the market you want to tap into, so you may want to say how you went about finding your information.

Local knowledge is a valid form of exploring the market. *(38)*

The local market *(39)*

This section creates a fuller picture of the geography and economics of the area you intend to work in. It will enable your lender to visualize your working environment and whether you have situated yourself in a financially feasible situation.

Several factors will be involved:

- *Ease of access.* Do people have to get in a car to get to you or can they walk or take a bus there? Does the position of your clinic in some way make visiting you more desirable than going anywhere else? *(40)*
- *Are people locally able to afford your services?* Lenders need to see you situated in an area that can financially sustain you. *(41)*
- *Can the area sustain the growth of your clinic?* Is there anything happening locally that will ensure a steady or increased supply of patients? For example, a new housing estate or more offices being built. *(42)*

Positioning

This is your identity in the marketplace and is how your patients and competitors perceive your particular service. It is what your clinic provides that makes it different or more attractive than other clinics.

Ask the following questions of yourself:

- *What makes the services you provide unique? (43)*
- *How do you want you and your clinic's services to be viewed? (44)*

These are questions you will be able to answer because of your market research.

Competitors

This is where you will have to differentiate your business from those of your competitors. Although you will not be required to name them, the lender may need a comparison of you and a selection of up to three competitors, under various headings such as:

- *Reputation.* It is very realistic to state that your competitor may have established a very good reputation. *(45)*
- *Location.* Has your location some advantage over the others? *(46)*
- *Service.* You will have to look at differentiating yourself on quality, price, hours of working, image, experience and capabilities of treatment. *(47)*

They do not need to be listed, but the following should be considered, as these questions may be asked by your lender to see if you appreciate the dynamics involved between you and your competitors.

- *What types of patient are your competitors going to treat successfully?*
- *What is each of your competitor's identity in the marketplace?*

Your lender may ask you for a SWOT analysis to see if you are aware of your *strengths, weaknesses, opportunities* and *threats.* Again, it is advisable to be honest or you will invalidate your other answers. Even if you are not required to present a brief SWOT analysis, the one you have prepared will help you not only with the business plan, but to know where you stand in the scheme of things.

You will be expected to have competitors and it will be a very unusual situation if you do not. Do consider any indirect competition. *(48)*

Pricing *(49)*

Again, this will be due to your market research. You do not want to be charging less than your competitors or your service may not be seen as credible, but you also do not want to charge more when starting out or you may put people off because you are too expensive.

Have a good explanation ready as to how you have set your price, although generally it is likely to be close to those of your competitors. Your price may be higher than those of your competitors, because you feel that your USP warrants a higher price.

Products may be a very small part of the pricing structure, but be ready if you are taking substantial stock on board to explain your pricing structure there.

Many herbalists use a prescription service, which may make the prescription a slightly higher price than that of competitors who do their own dispensing. You will need to explain that this removes the problem of stock, which can be very expensive, and that you can use the time spent dispensing for other more useful things, such as more treatments or time spent promoting yourself.

Customer profile

Be accurate and specific when describing your target patients. Generalization is not looked upon favourably, since it will seem you do not understand the type of patient you want to be treating.

Talk about their characteristics. You will need to consider the following:

- *Type.* Student, young professional, housewife, clerk. *(50)*
- *Age.* The age groups: young, old, teenager, retired. *(51)*
- *Gender.* A mixture or a predominant gender. *(52)*
- *Disposable income.* Readily available, moderate, limited. *(53)*
- *Location.* Where are your customers coming from – locally or further away? You have already included information regarding detailed geography in the introduction and local market sections. *(38–42)* This adds to the picture. *(54)*
- *The reasons why people should choose you as a therapist.* Experience, specialization, convenience, price. *(55)*
- *How regularly patients will be seeing you.* One-off visit, series of visits, checkups. *(56)*
- *What you are able to do for them. (57)*

There may be some overlap between this section and market size and trends.

Market size and trends

This indicates how much of the market you intend to capture and adds more detail to the market picture.

- *How many customers are available to your business?* You have largely covered this but may need to make a brief statement to fit in with the rest of this section. *(58)*
- *Where are you situated and what is its relevance to your practice?* You have already covered your precise location and its relevance to you in your business description. *(27, 29)* By now, potential lenders will have a reasonable idea of where you will be situated and its implications for you, but they will then need to know whether you are aiming for a local market or further away, and if the latter, how far away. *(59)*
- *Is the market in a growth or decline phase?* The economy may affect the amount of spare cash patients have available for private treatment. *(60)*
- *How are legal changes, registration going to affect your business?* Would such changes have a positive or negative impact on your therapy? Be honest. Making working practice difficult is not necessarily a bad thing as it may reduce less-qualified competition by making demands on

them they cannot meet. New legislation in the workplace may make businesses proactive in seeking ways to improve their employees' state of mind and health, by means of conservative treatments, such as complementary therapy. *(61)*

- *Is there a repeat demand for your service?* In some cases therapists may require to see patients for a series of treatments, in which case they should be able to accumulate a steady build-up of income. If this is not the case, it may be necessary to give more detail as to how you are going to sustain your income. This may be covered elsewhere in your market section, possibly in the customer profile section. *(62)*
- *Are you actively excluding any particular part of the market and why?* It is also acceptable to talk about the type of patients you will not be likely to attract to your clinic or whom you do not feel it is appropriate to treat. *(63)*

Some of the factors in Customer profile will overlap into this section and other areas of the business plan.

You must wherever possible cite sources for your statements.

Promotion strategy

You have already defined:

- The service you are providing (Product).
- Your market.
- Where you are in the market (Positioning).
- Your competition.
- Your pricing structure.
- Your target customer.

These all need to be brought together for your sales and marketing strategy. You need to show how you will draw patients into your clinic.

This should be concise and include:

- *How you intend to advertise.* You should describe all the methods you will use for your advertising, e.g. newspapers, fliers, advertising banners, and where you intend to place them. *(64)*
- *Whether you will be focusing your marketing within a certain area.* If so, where? *(65)*
- *Whether you have any useful contacts.* You may know someone on local radio or at a newspaper who could do an article on you.
- *Whether your profession is actively engaged in nationwide publicity.* Cited examples of this will be useful and are easily available from your professional body. *(66)*

This shows how you intend to make the public aware of your existence and the service you provide.

Have an example on A4 paper to demonstrate the appearance of your advertising, since this will give your lender a good idea of the image you are trying to convey.

Contact your professional body to see if they can send you examples of the literature you can buy from them. Some associations supply a certain amount of leaflets free of charge every time you renew your membership.

This is a good time to stress that you belong to a professional body and the effort they make on your behalf every year in PR. Many give a list with regular news mailings to show just how much PR activity they have engaged in over a particular period. This will be useful information to include for your lender. If your professional body employs a professional PR firm then do mention this. *(67)*

Your advertising costing should be included somewhere, with an idea of when large charges, e.g. telephone book advertising, are likely to be incurred, although these now can be paid off in instalments. Any exhibitions you will attend which require unusual expenditure should also be noted.

Financial considerations

This is where you pull together all the expenses incurred in running your business. These are the figures that back up what you have so far said in words.

A lender is largely concerned with cash flow, which in the complementary profession is good, as the payment is usually instantaneous for the service.

A lender will look at your financial section to ascertain several things.

- *Can you repay your loan?*
- *What is your profitability?*
- *Are you able to cover your interest payments?*
- *If security of the loan is required, do you have any that can be used?* This is usually your home, but is only required on a large loan.

The calculations will be summaries of the following:

- Operating expenses.
- Capital requirements.
- Cost of goods.

Operating expenses. These include marketing, and overheads. Your overheads include fixed expenses such as administrative costs, and other expenses that remain constant regardless of how busy your practice gets, such as utilities, cleaning, wages, etc. Overheads also include such things as travel, equipment, hire purchase, leasing and supplies.

Capital requirements. These detail the amount of money you will need to buy your equipment, for example couches, vacuum cleaners, kettles, etc., in order to start up and continue practising.

Cost of goods. Ideally these should only be a very small consideration when setting up, unless you are a herbalist and want a pharmacy, in which case the amount may be considerable. Work out what you need and err on the side of too much rather than too little, but keep it within sensible limits.

You will need to have an idea of how much you will use a year. Your clinical practice module is a good time to assess just how much stock you will need and its turnover.

All these considerations enable you to put together the following, which must be presented to the lender:

- Profit and loss forecast
- Cash-flow statement
- Income statement.

Do make sure that they are presented in an easily understood format. Lenders spend a great deal of time examining dozens of applications a week for loans. An easily understood format not only makes it much easier for them to follow your financial calculations, but will also make them feel more comfortable about the proposal you have put in front of them.

Estimated sales

As you will have discovered from the financial introduction chapter (Ch. 15), this is always a difficult area for assessment.

Estimates should be based on the numbers of potential customers you have in your area.

Certain statistics relevant to the economy nationally can be viewed on the Office for National Statistics website (see p. 220).

Your type of therapy makes a great deal of difference to the number of visits a patient is likely to make. Chiropractors and osteopaths tend to achieve a higher number of repeat visits because their services are often needed as a result of trauma and the need to return to work as quickly as possible. Patients seeking homeopathic treatment often have a more chronic problem and less urgency to seek treatment; therefore patient availability may be less. Different therapists also take a different length of time for each treatment and logically there can only be so many patients that a practitioner can accommodate in a working day.

Do not be too optimistic about sales and profit margins.

Do give reasons for the assumptions on growth you have made.

Profit and loss forecast

This is a summary of your business transactions for a given period, which will be 12 months. You will deduct total expenditure from total income, to show whether your business will make a profit or loss at the end of the period you have chosen.

Do not worry if your business is not making a large profit by the end of the first year. It is usual to take up to 3 years to start to see some suitable profit being made and your lender will expect this.

The lender needs to see a steady growth in your business and the attainment of a profit within a suitable period of time.

Once you have your loan it is important to keep producing a profit/loss account, which is usually done by your accountant. If you are classed as self-employed and require a mortgage or another loan you need to provide accounts for 3 years. The profit/loss account will be part of the consideration.

Cash-flow and profit/loss forecast

This shows:

- How much money you will need.
- When you will need it.
- Where the money will come from.

It demonstrates month by month how the cash is moving in and out of your business.

Since it gives you a monthly picture, the cash-flow statement will give you the ability to make sensible business decisions and act to warn you if your expenditure is getting out of hand. This will enable you to work out ways to deal with the situation before it gets out of hand, by economizing or cutting back on spending.

The cash-flow forecast shows both you and your lender how much money is needed to keep the business running (working capital).

Before you submit the financial documents, do the following:

- *Make sure that all your figures can be reconciled.* Your lender will check your calculations thoroughly.
- *Have an accountant check over your financial calculations.* This will ensure that all the figures can be reconciled.
- *Avoid an unrealistic build-up in your business.* You do not want to be overoptimistic, then have to explain to your lender why you are running into trouble.
- *Do not underestimate your requirements.*

Income statement

This is where you explain your case for your ability to generate cash. You will record:

- Income.
- Expenses.
- Capital.
- Cost of goods.

All of these together will demonstrate how much money you will make or lose in that year. This should be done month by month.

It is very likely the lender will want to know how you decided on the numbers for your predictions of patients. Use only a short summary to justify your predictions. For example, you may have worked in a clinic where you knew the standard throughput, or talked to experienced practitioners about their start-up, or you may have been able to talk to one of the practitioners in the area.

Conclusion

Producing a business plan is a worthwhile exercise regardless of how small a loan you will need or if you need one at all.

When producing a business plan for a lender, do not cut corners. It is important to work out every aspect of it very carefully.

Be able to back up the statements you make.

Do get someone, if possible your accountant, to reconcile your calculations as mistakes can ruin your credibility.

Above all, do be honest in your appraisal as it will be of benefit to you in the long term.

Useful websites

Australia

http://www.abs.gov.au/

Australian Bureau of Statistics

http://www.auda.org.au/domains/au-domains/

Australian Domain Name Adminstrator
Information about registering domain name.

Business name registration
https://bizline.docep.wa.gov.au/bnonline/

Western Australia

http://www.business.act.gov.au/businesslicences/business_name_registration

Australian Central Government

http://www.consumer.qld.gov.au/oft/oftweb.nsf/web+pages/86A22C693B42F48E4A256E1B001A251A?OpenDocument

Queensland

http://www.consumer.tas.gov.au/forms#business%20names

Tasmania

http://blis.fairtrading.nsw.gov.au/businessnames/registeringabusinessname.html

New South Wales

http://www.nt.gov.au/justice/graphpages/cba/docs/ba_bn_f1_appn_206.pdf

Northern Territory Government

http://www.ocba.sa.gov.au/assets/files/01_App_reg_bus_name.pdf

South Australia

http://online.justice.vic.gov.au/servlet/cav_home

Victoria

Canada

Many websites are bilingual.

http://bsa.cbsc.org/gol/bsa/site.nsf/en/su04914.html

Canadian Government Business Startup
Follow the links for the various provinces or territories to find information on business names and registration.

http://www12.statcan.ca/english/census01/home/index.cfm

Census of Canada

New Zealand

Governmental websites are bilingual.

http://www.companies.govt.nz/pls/web/dbssiten.main

New Zealand Government
Companies site to register your business name if you are forming a company.

http://www.iponz.govt.nz/pls/web/dbssiten.main

Intellectual Property Office of New Zealand
Site for registering a trademark.

UK

http://wck2.companieshouse.gov.uk

Companies House

http://www.nic.uk

Nominet

http://www.start.biz/home.htm

National Business Register

http://www.statistics.gov.uk/

Office for National Statistics

USA

http://www.census.gov/

United States Census Bureau

http://www.nic.us/

NeuStar
US Registry operator for US domain name registration.

http://www.uspto.gov/index.html

United States Patent and Trademark Office
If you have a logo that is unique and brands your business distinctively.

Business name registration

The procedure for registering a business name can vary from state to state. Usually the name is registered at a county level. Probably the best action is to call your county clerk's office for more information.

Appendix

BUSINESS PLAN *(1)*
WESTSIDE CHIROPRACTIC CLINIC *(2)*

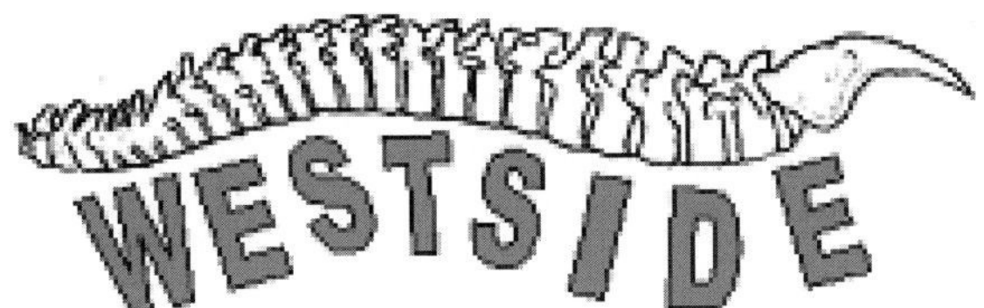

(3)

J M SMITH *(2)*
25 The Street *(4)*
Anytown
Countyshire
Telephone 01111 578659 *(5)*
westchiro@pelican.com *(6)*

16 September 2005 *(7)*

Executive summary

Introduction

I intend to open the Westside Chiropractic Clinic in three months' time. *(8)* The short-term financial goal of the clinic is to become financially self-sufficient within two years, enabling me to work there full time. The long-term goal of the clinic is to become a centre of excellence within the community for family-orientated chiropractic treatment *(9)* and associated therapies. Able to expand on its intended site and with the option of buying the premises it will be renting, it is ideally situated to fulfil this goal.

Business description

The clinic will be housed in an annexe to the local pharmacy. The site has good off-road parking, with plenty of on-street parking close by. It is in the middle of a thriving shopping centre, on one of the main roads into town. Local transport is efficient and frequent. *(10)*

I will be the proprietor. I have an MSc in chiropractic, and am a registered chiropractor. I have three years' clinical experience as an undergraduate at the college clinic and two years' postgraduate experience at the Othercity Chiropractic Clinic in Othercity. *(11)*

The services

Chiropractic treatment is manipulative therapy that can be delivered, with appropriate modifications, to any age group.

It can be used successfully to treat back and neck pain, sports injuries, and limb pain. It is also accepted as being able to help headaches, migraines and infant colic. *(9)*

The clinic will have two late-night openings a week and will also open on two Saturday mornings a month.

The market

The clinic is situated in a highly sought after area of professional people, who will actively seek private treatment such as chiropractic to reduce time off work. *(12)*

The area is largely inhabited by families because of its schools and large properties and is advertised as such in literature for house sales. More housing is currently being planned.

The Westside district has a population of approximately 90,000, with an employment rate higher than the national average.

There is also potential for out of town trade as there is very little in the way of similar treatment available in the outlying districts and, with traffic in the centre of town being discouraged, the area where the clinic is due to be sited is well patronized, as it is convenient to get to and parking is not a problem. It is also on a main bus route into town. *(13)*

Competitive advantage

There are several clinics in and around the city offering similar services. These include other chiropractors, osteopaths and physiotherapists.

There is only one clinic within a mile of the intended site, which is a chiropractic clinic. Most of the other clinics are sited on the other side of the city.

The Westside Chiropractic Clinic will be situated in the heart of a residential area in the main shopping centre. There is easy access and good parking, and patients will be more inclined to make use of a service that is on their doorstep and is easy to get to. *(12)*

The clinic is also sited on the main shopping thoroughfare, so patients from out of town will see it as an easy opportunity to complete their purchases and get treated without having to make separate trips.

Being associated with the pharmacy will be very helpful, since it is to their benefit financially to promote the clinic, both short term and long term.

No one as yet has focused on the family as a target group. Only three similar clinics currently offer extended working hours.

Marketing strategy *(14)*

As the clinic is likely to attract customers walking by, there will be advertising on display in the windows and in the pharmacy.

While the clinic is starting up, there will always be someone on reception, even when the chiropractor is not there to answer calls and queries.

Yellow Pages advertising, as well as local magazine advertising will be heavily utilized.

Open days will be held to encourage people into the clinic to discuss chiropractic treatment, and free screenings will be available to anyone who is not sure chiropractic treatment suits their needs.

Talks have been arranged with local groups.

Special clinics will be run to encourage parents to bring children and babies into the clinic.

Summary of financial projections and financial requirements *(15, 16)*

	First year	**Second year**	**Third year**
			Assuming income/overhead/living remain the same
	52,650	104,300	104,300
Overheads including purchase of equipment and £28,800 living expenses	78,662	75,415	75,415
Profit/shortfall	–26,012	28,885	
Deduct shortfall from year 1		26,012	
Net profit year 2		2873	
Net profit year 3			28,885

The maximum borrowing in the first year would be £28,904
Year 3 is to demonstrate that if income/overhead and living expenses remain as year 2 the net profit for year 3 increases dramatically due to clearing the debt in year 2.

Table of contents *(17)*

The industry

At any one time 33% of people will be experiencing back pain. 80% of the adult population will suffer significant back pain at some point in their lives. Businesses lose 4.9 million working days a year due to work-related back pain (TUC). *(18)*

Chiropractic is one of the leading complementary therapies. It has been providing healthcare treatment since 1895.

The National Chiropractic Association was established in 1930 and 70% of all chiropractors in the country belong to this association. *(19)*

There are currently just over 2000 registered chiropractors in the country. *(20)*

Both the National Chiropractic Association and the Chiropractic Register work to promote chiropractic as well as maintain a high professional standard amongst registered chiropractors. There is a strict code of ethics and a requirement to conduct continual postgraduate education. *(21)*

Since 2001 the title chiropractor has been protected by law and it is now a criminal offence for anyone to describe themselves as a chiropractor if they are not registered with the statutory, regulatory body, the General Chiropractic Council, established by the Chiropractors Act 1994 (GCC). *(22)*

There is currently growth in the profession as public awareness continues to grow and research conducted within the chiropractic profession improves its standing with the orthodox medical profession. *(23)*

A recent clinical trial involving manipulation found that 'spinal manipulation is a cost-effective addition to "best care" for back pain in general practice.' (UKBEAM). *(24)*

Trades Union Congress (TUC): www.tuc.org.uk
General Chiropractic Council (GCC): www.gcc-uk.org
UK BEAM Trial Team 2004 United Kingdom Back Pain, Exercise and Manipulation (UK/BEAM) Randomised Trial Effectiveness of Physical Treatment for Back Pain in Primary Care. BMJ 329(7479): 1377

Business description

The Westside Chiropractic Clinic, *(25)* due to open in three months' time, will be located in one of the most sought after districts in Anytown. Sited next door to the Market Street Pharmacy and on the main thoroughfare of Suburb, it is well placed to become a prominent centre for chiropractic care. *(26)*

The Westside Chiropractic Clinic will be situated in a newly refurbished suite of rooms in an annexe adjoining the pharmacy. The rooms have a separate entrance and are independent of the pharmacy. The owner of the Market Street Pharmacy is also the landlord, and is an enthusiastic supporter of complementary therapy. The pharmacy currently stocks a range of homeopathic and herbal remedies, and sees the establishment of a reputable complementary therapist as a positive and logical extension of the pharmacy. The work currently being done is due to be finished within the next eight weeks. *(27)*

Anytown is a university city with a population of 270,000. Its main industries are pharmaceutical production, technology and administration.

The Westside district has a population of approximately 90,000. This comprises 18% retired people, 22% between the ages of 45 years and retirement, and 37% 16- to 45-year-olds. The employment rate is higher than the national average. *(28)*

Market Street is part of a well-patronized shopping area with a mixture of grocers, baker, butcher and bespoke home decoration shops and a small art gallery. There are also a variety of small restaurants with a delicatessen that has a small coffee shop attached.

There is considerable passing trade as it is a main route into the city. There is also a good bus service, with buses passing every few minutes, and the nearest bus stop is a few metres down from the pharmacy. There is a generous amount of off-street parking due to the anticipation of the owner of the pharmacy that this would be a requirement of a clinic. There is also easy parking down the various side roads from the main road. *(29)*

Statistics from the Office for National Statistics website:
http://neighbourhood.statistics.gov.uk/dissemination/

Objectives (30)

Short term

- *Financial.* To reach a break-even point within two years.
- *Business.* To be able to run the clinic full time in two years.

Long term

- *Financial.* To build up to maximum patient load in three years with a view to buying premises.
- *Business.* To be able to establish a multidisciplinary practice within five years.

The clinic

Mission statement *(31)*

The mission of the Westside Chiropractic Clinic is to provide convenient, high-quality, and affordable chiropractic treatment focusing on community and family care.

The nature of the clinic

As well as treating general spinal conditions such as back and neck pain, a chiropractor will also treat a variety of injuries or conditions of the limbs. *(32)*

Other conditions, not immediately linked with chiropractic treatment, such as headaches, migraines, asthma or infant colic, may be improved with chiropractic care (GCC).

I intend opening within three months pending final completion of building work to the annexe. *(33)*

Ownership and management *(34)*

I will be sole proprietor of the clinic and therefore its principal.

Having completed a five-year full-time MSc in Chiropractic at the College of Chiropractic in Seatown, where I received a year's clinical training, I went on to work at the Othercity Chiropractic Clinic in Othercity. I have been working there for the last two years.

During this time I have taken courses in paediatric chiropractic treatment with a view to encouraging the chiropractic treatment of children and babies.

A requirement of my degree was to write a thesis in which I examined the benefits of chiropractic care given to family groups and whether establishing a family-orientated practice was a worthwhile enterprise.

I have deliberately sought to establish a clinic in an area that is known to be family orientated.

I am a member of the National Chiropractic Association and a registered chiropractor.

I will be working part time, three to three and a half days a week, at my own clinic while continuing to work two days at the Othercity Chiropractic Clinic. In the second year my days at my own clinic will increase to four, and by the third year I will be working there full time.

My colleagues in the Othercity Chiropractic Clinic have been made fully aware of my plans.

Staff (35)

My receptionist has lived all her life in Anytown and until her recent retirement was a receptionist at a local surgery. She has received complementary treatment in one form or other for most of her life. She is involved in the local Women's Institute. She enjoyed her work as a doctor's receptionist and sees the new clinic as an exciting new project to be involved in.

I am fortunate enough to have several relatives in the area, including my parents who are retired, who are keen to help me in my new project. Their contacts in the local community will prove invaluable in building links into the community.

Description of services

I will deliver treatment consisting of a combination of manipulative treatment where applicable and appropriate management advice.

My treatment time will also include advice on diet and lifestyle to encompass not only the patient, but hopefully engage the whole family unit. *(36)*

I expect to treat a wide age range, but will encourage both the young and elderly as this is an area in the population for which there is very little provision. (36)

It is my intention to introduce a half-day session every month at a reduced rate, where I will screen the children and infants of the parents I currently treat, to introduce them to the concept of chiropractic care at an early age.

Chiropractic treatment will be provided initially three days a week, with two late nights and a Saturday morning clinic every two weeks, to accommodate family members who might find difficulty in attending daytime appointments. (37)

The market

Introduction

My market research has been conducted using local statistical resources on the Internet and by personal assessment of the local area. I have also talked extensively to local business about setting up a clinic.

The pharmacist in whose premises I intend to work has a chain of pharmacies in the surrounding county and has previously rented to chiropractors and osteopaths, who are successfully running their own clinics from similar annexes to that of the pharmacy. The insights I have gained from talking to them have been invaluable.

As a native of Anytown, I have a good understanding of the geography, economics and people of the area. *(38)*

The local market *(39)*

The clinic will be providing chiropractic treatment for inhabitants in the immediate vicinity of the local area. Many of the residents are within walking distance and generally tend to make good use of the local facilities, which provide for most of their needs without them having to venture too far from home. The clinic should make a welcome addition to the locality, and its location will be one of the important factors in its success. The parking restrictions in the city and volume of traffic at most times of the day discourage extensive travelling into the city unless it is for work or a special occasion. *(40)*

The area in which the clinic will be situated is a highly sought after district with house prices in the range of £160,000 at the lower end of the market, rising to £300,000. The local state schools, both primary and secondary, have a higher than national average for academic achievement. Families largely inhabit the area. There is some student accommodation in the area, but the main student housing is on the other side of the city along with the university campus. *(41)*

Planning permission has just been obtained for new executive-style housing on the outskirts of the district. (42)

Positioning

There are very few practitioners who target the very young and the very old *(43)* and with this in mind it is my intention to create a practice where family groups are encouraged and the clinic is seen to be as important an element of the community as the pharmacy. *(44)*

Competitors

There are currently eight chiropractors working in Anytown. Four of these work in well-established clinics, while the other four have been open between a year and 18 months. *(45)*

The majority of these clinics are on the east side of the city, because of the high cost of setting up on the more desirable west side.

Only three chiropractors currently work on the west side of the city, in the same clinic and within two miles of the intended location of Westside Chiropractic Clinic.

The possibility of expansion for that particular clinic is severely limited and possibilities of relocation in that area are also limited.

The chiropractor in the city centre generally only sees patients who arrive on public transport or on foot, as parking in the city centre is difficult. There is no room for expansion in that location.

The Westside Chiropractic Clinic is well positioned to attract passing trade, as it will be located right in the heart of the community on a busy pedestrian and traffic thoroughfare, with ample off-road parking. The pharmacy is the only one in this suburb and forms a vital link with the community. The close association with it should benefit the clinic.

There is currently room on the site for expansion, for which planning permission has been given, and as an option to buy is a possibility in the future, the clinic would not need to move in order to enlarge. *(46)*

Three clinics offer late-night appointments and appointments on Saturday mornings. The closest clinic rotates the responsibility between its three chiropractors. *(47)*

There are also eight osteopaths and ten physiotherapists in the city, only one of which works from a pharmacy in a situation similar to the one that I propose, and about a mile away from where I plan to run my business. *(48)*

Pricing *(49)*

The treatment charge of £26 is slightly higher than the average fee for chiropractic treatment for Anytown, but is comparable with the nearest clinic on this side of the city, where prices for services are generally higher. The accessibility of the clinic should also encourage patients to use its services.

The mother and baby clinic will have a nominal charge of £5 on the basis that the time spent is a form of PR, as well as encouraging the idea of the importance of spinal health at any age.

Customer profile

The clinic will be at the heart of a residential community of largely professional people. *(50)* Most patients will be on average between 30 and 60 years of age (approximately 60% of the local population) *(51)* and a relatively even mixture of males and females. *(52)*

Most of the houses in this location are three- to four-bedroom family houses. There are two primary schools, a large state secondary school and a private school.

The street the clinic will be located on has remained the busiest and most commercially stable for the last five years. *(53)*

Although most of the patients visiting the clinic will be drawn from the local community within a radius of approximately two miles, because of its ease of access from the motorway and ring road, ease of parking and its location on a main bus route, patients living as far a ten miles away could be encouraged to use its services. *(54, 55, 59)*

Because opening hours extend beyond normal working hours, there is a possibility of picking up patients on their way home, and Saturday openings are also likely to encourage patients who have difficultly visiting on a weekday. *(55, 56)*

Patients are expected to attend for a minimum of six visits, and check-ups every two months will be encouraged to maintain or limit their presenting condition. *(56, 57, 62)*

Market size and trends

Since a sizeable proportion of the local population are professional people between 30 and 60 years old (60% of the local population), *(58)* there is considerable disposable income, as indicated by the price and type of merchandise available in shops in the main shopping area and the care that has been taken to maintain the shops. *(53)*

Currently, with absenteeism from work, and the health service waiting list increasing, private treatment such as chiropractic is being sought to deal with injuries that if left long term could become a chronic problem. Private healthcare is becoming an acceptable fact of life, with many people choosing to take out some type of healthcare policy in order to receive rapid attention to any medical problem that may occur. There are now many companies who openly advertise complementary therapy as one of the services they will pay for. *(60)*

Most health insurance companies are more confident since the registration of chiropractic that there is adequate accountability within the profession. Many of the local residents work for large national firms, who routinely provide private healthcare for their employees. (61)

I am not actively excluding any particular group of patients from receiving my treatment, but having seen practices where the community and family aspect is embraced, I know that this method of conducting a clinic leads to a steady referral rate via word of mouth. (63)

Advertising and promotion

Several methods of advertising will be used: *(64)* Yellow Pages; window advertisements; posters and leaflets to be delivered to selected local shops; initial advertisement in local newspaper to advertise opening with an associated editorial; and the Parish Magazine. *(65)*

The clinic is timed to open a month before the Yellow Pages for the area comes out. *(65)*

Posters in the window should interest passing trade, and my receptionist will be there some of the day when I am not there to answer questions and take bookings over the phone. Relatives have volunteered to cover the rest of the time to perform the same function. *(65)*

The pharmacy will display my poster and keep my professional body's leaflets by the counter. Before the clinic opens, all the staff will have attended a small seminar on the benefits of chiropractic. *(65)*

Financial considerations

Assumptions and build-up of overheads

Services	**£34,251**			
First month		**Last month**		
Insurance for boiler	180	Servicing equipment	168	
Electrical testing	72	Basic month cost	2568	
Registration of business name	60		2736	
Data protection	35	Basic third month	276	
Line monitoring	396	Total last month	3012	
Business insurance	900			
Vehicle insurance	400			
Road fund licence	120			
	2163	**Basic month**		
Add basic cost of month	2568	Wages plus		
Total first month	4731	service		£34,251
		Deduct		
		First month	2163	
		Last month	168	
		Sharps	48	
		Water	456	

Electricity	300	
Gas	300	
	3435	3435
		30,816

Every third month				
Basic month cost		2568		
Sharps	48			
Water	456			
Gas	300		Divide by 12 months	£2568 pcm
Electricity	300			
	1104			
Divided by 4 =		276		
		2844 pcm		

First month		**4731**
Months 2, 4, 5, 7, 8, 10, 11 =	7 × 2568	17,976
Months 3, 6, 9 =	3 × 2844	8532
Last month		3012
		£34,251

Advertising **£3390**

First month			Basic month	
Yellow Pages*	1300		Total for advertising	3390
Professional leaflets	90		Deduct first month	1390
	1390			2000
Monthly charge	167			
	1557		Divided by 12 months, say	167
			2–12 @ £167	
Months				
2–12 = 11 @ £167	1837			
	£3394	Differential is in monthly calculation		

*Need to find out timing of advertisement in Yellow Pages, as the publication may be part way through the financial year

Stationery **£2132**

		Total stationery	£2132
		Renewable every 3 months	
		Therefore divide by 4	£533
Months 1, 4, 7, 10 =	£533		
4 × 533 =	£2132		

Equipment — **£3065 initial cost + £574 depreciation per year**
Total £3639

First month			Monthly charge	
Assume all equipment bought in first month			Depreciation	£574
Total cost plus depreciation	3065		Divided by 12 months, say	£48 pcm
	48			
	3113			
Months				
2–12 = 11 × 48	528			
	£3641	Differential is in monthly calculation		

Professional fees — **£4900**

First month		Monthly charge	
Register membership	1000	Seminars	2000
Professional membership	900	Accountant balance	400
Accountant (part)	200		2400
Solicitor	400		
Monthly charge	200	Divided by 12 months =	£200 pcm
	2700		

Months 2–12 = 11 × £200	2200		
	£4900		

Consumables	**£1338**		
Months			
1, 3, 5, 7, 9, 11		Total consumables	£1338
6 × £223 =	£1338	Renewable every 2 months	
		Therefore £1338 divided	
		by 6 = £223	

Sundries	**£170 + £34 depreciation per year**	
First month	**Total £204**	
Assume all sundries bought in first month Months 2–12 @ £3 pcm		Depreciation £34
Monthly charge	170	Divided by 12 months, say £3 pcm
	3	
First month	173	
Months 2–12 = 11 × £3 pcm	33	
	£ 206	Differential is in monthly calculation

Cash-flow and profit/loss forecast

First year

Month	1	2	3	4	5	6	7	8	9	10	11	12	
Services	4731	2568	2844	2568	2568	2844	2568	2568	2844	2568	2568	3012	
Advertising	1557	167	167	167	167	167	167	167	167	167	167	167	
Stationery	533			533			533			533			
Equipment	3113	48	48	48	48	48	48	48	48	48	48	48	
Professional fees	2700	200	200	200	200	200	200	200	200	200	200	200	
Consumables	223		223		223		223		223		223		
Sundries	173	3	3	3	3	3	3	3	3	3	3	3	
Total	13,030	2986	3485	3519	3209	3262	3742	2986	3485	3519	3209	3430	49,862
Living expenses	2400	2400	2400	2400	2400	2400	2400	2400	2400	2400	2400	2400	28,800
Total	15,430	5386	5885	5919	5609	5662	6142	5386	5885	5919	5609	5830	
Income (Incl. other clinic)	500	1800	3700	4200	3500	5100	5600	3050	4950	7100	7600	5550	52,650
Monthly ±	–14,930	–3586	–2185	–1719	–2109	–562	–542	–2336	–935	1181	1991	–280	
Cum ±		–18,516	–20,701	–22,420	–24,529	–25,091	–25,633	–27,969	–28,904	–27,723	–25,732	–26,012	c/fwd

Overdraft interest depending on amount could add £2000 to £26,268 loan

Second year

Assuming overheads and living expenses (less initial cost of equipment and sundries) are as first year, and income basis as per monthly schedule

Total	12,183	5386	5885	5919	5609	5662	6142	5386	5885	5919	5609	5830	75,415
Income	7200	10,100	10,100	10,100	7200	10,100	10,100	4800	7200	10,100	10,100	7200	104,300
Monthly ±	–4983	4714	4215	4181	1591	4438	3958	–586	1315	4181	4491	1370	
Cum b/fwd	–26,012												
Cum ±	30,995	–26,281	–22,066	–17,885	–16,294	–11,856	–7898	–8484	–7169	–2988	1503	2873	

The Parish Magazine is seen as an important newsletter and comes out once a month. The advertising cost is very minimal for a year. *(65)*

As a public relations exercise, the clinic will have an open day where I will give talks at set times during the day. Local groups such as women's groups and self-help groups have been contacted for talks over the next few months. *(65)*

Free screenings will be made available to potential patients if they are not sure whether chiropractic is appropriate for their condition. *(65)*

The National Chiropractic Association have been very helpful in giving advertising and general PR advice and employ a professional PR company to assist them in raising awareness of chiropractic at a national level. *(66, 67)*

Sales projections

My sales projections are based on the following assumptions. The local population will wish to return to work after injury as soon as possible. They have the means, either as disposable income or medical insurance policies, to have access to private medicine, which assures them of rapid access to treatment.

Having already worked at a clinic where I had to build up a patient load, and after conversations with colleagues in similar situations, I feel confident that I am going to be able to accurately assess the build-up of patients.

Assumptions and build-up of income

First year

Month	Holidays (weeks)	Days worked	Patients		Patients		Amount (£)	Total (£)
			New	Rate	Repeat	Rate		
1	1	12	4	£50			200	
					12	£25	300	500
2		16	16	£50			800	
					40	£25	1000	1800
3		16	18	£50			900	
					112	£25	2800	3700
4		16	20	£50			1000	
					128	£25	3200	4200
5	1	12	16	£50			800	
					108	£25	2700	3500
6		16	22	£50			1100	
					160	£25	4000	5100
7		16	24	£50			1200	
					176	£25	4400	5600
8	2	8	13	£50			650	
					96	£25	2400	3050
9	1	12	21	£50			1050	
					156	£25	3900	4950
10		16	30	£50			1500	
					224	£25	5600	7100
11		16	32	£50			1600	
					240	£25	6000	7600
12	1	12	21	£50			1050	
					180	£25	4500	5550
								52,650

Second year

Income per month based on the following – 3 new patients per day + 18 repeat patients per day

16 days × 3 = 58 patients × £50 = £2900
16 days × 18 = 288 patients × £25 = £7200
Therefore 16-day month = £10,100

8 days × 3 = 24 patients × £50 = £1200
8 days × 18 = 144 patients × £25 = £3600
Therefore 8-day month = £4800

12 days × 3 = 36 patients × £50 = £1800
12 days × 18 = 216 patients × £25 = £5400
Therefore 12-day month = £7200

Month	Holidays (weeks)	Days worked	Income per month
1	1	12	7200
2		16	10,100
3		16	10,100
4		16	10,100
5	1	12	7200
6		16	10,100
7		16	10,100
8	2	8	4800
9	1	12	7200
10		16	10,100
11		16	10,100
12	1	12	7200
			104,300

Income statement

I intend to continue working at Othercity Chiropractic Clinic for the next two years on a part-time basis. The first year I will work two days a week seeing on average 25 patients each day. In the second year this will drop to one day a week. It is my intention by year three to be financially self-sufficient.

I have been able to build up a working capital of £5000.

Revenue projections

	First year	Second year	Third year
			Assuming income/overhead/living remain the same
	52,650	104,300	104,300
Overheads including purchase of equipment and £28,800 living expenses	78,662	75,415	75,415
Profit/shortfall	–26,012	28,885	
Deduct shortfall from year 1		26,012	
Net profit year 2		2873	
Net profit year 3			28,885

The maximum borrowing in the first year would be £28,904
Year 3 is to demonstrate that if income/overhead and living expenses remain as year 2 the net profit for year 3 increases dramatically due to clearing the debt in year 2.

Organizing finance 18

Chapter contents

Raising money

It is very unusual for a practitioner not to need money to set up a new clinic. At the very least you will need to give the room you will be working in an air of professionalism, which may require the renovation of furniture or basic decoration to freshen it up. You will also need business cards and some promotional literature.

The amount of money you will require will vary considerably depending on how ambitiously you want to start. Working from home and from a licensed premises are probably the most cost-effective ways to start, requiring only a minimum outlay of cash.

Having worked through your finances, you will have a good idea of how much cash you will be able to generate per year and what your shortfall is likely to be. As long as the shortfall is a temporary situation, then you will need to look at a loan, largely to cover your start-up expenses. So where do you get your money from? There are several ways this can be approached.

Do you have anything you can sell?

Your car may be too large for your needs. Is it possible to sell it and run a smaller one that is less expensive to maintain? The moderate amount of money you will make from this transaction may go some way towards the set-up cost. Downsizing will also be financially beneficial in the long term.

Do you own anything of value such as antiques or jewellery? This is a variable market, but again some of the money you make can go towards the cost of your new clinic.

Borrowing from relatives or friends

This is not an ideal situation unless you have a very understanding relationship. If you encounter financial problems they may never see the money again or it may take a long time for them to recover it.

It may also involve the need for them to feel that they have a right to interfere with the running of your business. Any investment they may make in your business has to be done with the understanding that they leave you to make your own decisions, and this situation relies on a great deal of trust and faith from your lenders.

Banks

Although banks do give unsecured loans, it is unlikely you will be given one without producing some sort of justification for its requirement. A business plan will more than likely be needed to show you have thought things through and understand every aspect of your business, particularly the financial elements.

Beyond a certain limit the bank, as with any lender, will require a loan to be secured against your home. The deeds of the property may have to be handed to the bank. This may then mean that you will be doubly in debt, not only to the bank, but also to the lender of your mortgage if you have one.

It is a good idea to ask about overdraft and loan facilities, including the interest rate you will be paying above base, and the degree of security required. Obtaining a promise not to call in the loan without notice is also advisable. The size of overdraft the bank is likely to give may also be a deciding factor.

Banks are open to negotiation and it may be possible to haggle over the interest rate on your loan, before you take it out. This does, however, require a good grasp of interest rates and loans, so it may be worth talking the deal over with your accountant, who can advise you.

There are other forms of security, which may come from a life policy or stocks and shares, but your home is a more usual request for security.

It may be possible to enlist a credible guarantor, which might be a relative or friend. A bank will rarely accept the guarantor as being able to cover the entire loan unless the person is very well known to that bank. The bank will probably ask for some security from the guarantor such as a life policy or stocks and shares.

Banks tend to be cautious and may not lend to potential borrowers who are unknown to them because they are not comfortable with the way they present themselves or their business plan. Above all, banks want figures and evidence of a logical thought process to back them.

An overdraft may be the most sensible option, as it does not require security. It is a way of having short-term finance in difficult cash-flow situations. It is not, however, the best way to borrow money since you will incur a set-up charge, a monthly administration charge and the interest on the account, but these can be set off against tax.

The interest charged will be linked to the bank base rate and will vary. Your overdraft will be reviewed every 12 months unless it seems to be spiralling out of control.

Short-term loans

These are usually a better option than hire purchase, but you may be able to get a better deal on hire purchase if you bargain. You may also not wish to borrow from one source but spread your payments around. If you do choose this method, you must have a very clear idea of when your payments go out and for exactly how much, or you will lose track of what you owe and have a tendency to overspend.

You may wish to go for a fixed rate of interest rather than a variable rate. A bank loan will mean that once you have bought your equipment it is yours rather than belonging to the hire purchase company until you have finished all the payments.

Medium-term loans

These may last up to 10 years and repayments are usually flexible in that they can be scheduled to suit the financial fluctuations that may occur in your business.

You might arrange to pay off parts of the loan at particular points in the year. It may also be possible to arrange a delay in the repayment until the first or second year of the loan. The downside is that the repayment will be higher later on to compensate for this 'honeymoon period'. This situation, however, would require a great deal of negotiation and may be considered unusual.

Long-term loans

These are over 10 years' duration and are usually for buying property.

Commercial mortgages

These are taken out for businesses and are usually for a shorter period than domestic mortgages, lasting only 10 to 15 years rather than 20 to 25 years. There is tax relief on this type of mortgage.

Many lenders offer 'repayment holidays'. Payments can be made monthly or quarterly and interest can be fixed or variable. Security for the finance is given by signing over the deeds of the property to the lender, so that if there is a default, lenders can quickly sell the property and reclaim their money.

Insurances such as life insurance may also have to be taken out and made out to the lender.

Hire purchase

Hire purchase enables you to buy large equipment straight away, without having to negotiate a loan from the bank, but the repayments will have to be included in your financial calculations.

Be careful to read the contract, however, as you might find that you do not actually own the equipment after you have finished paying for it. If this is the situation, you will retain the use of the equipment for a minimal fee, payable each year, usually by direct debit.

The repayment cost may also be higher than for a bank loan, but will ensure that you are not reliant on the bank for all your expenses, which is why this form of loan may be favoured.

Interest-free credit

Some firms sell their equipment by offering interest-free credit to lure you into buying from them. Providing you can afford the initial deposit and keep up the monthly payments or pay the outstanding money at the end of the credit period, this may be another way of buying equipment.

Credit cards

Using these will delay the payment for quite a few weeks if skilfully done. It will also be possible to pay in instalments; however, the interest rate on credit cards is high and using them is only preferable to an overdraft as a short-term option. Care has to be taken in spending this way since you can run the risk of placing yourself further in debt if you are tempted to buy something you have not budgeted for.

Second mortgage on the house

Compared to any other possession, your home is likely to be worth a substantial amount of money. This is not a quick way of raising money, however, and it is risky to tie your house so directly to your business. As someone who is self-employed and possibly not registered as a company, your personal assets are already at risk, since you may not have limited liability.

You are only likely to get a loan against the value of your house if the lender thinks you can afford the additional monthly repayments. If you have paid off only the interest on your mortgage and not the capital, then it is unlikely that you will be able to get a loan.

It may well be that you are not the sole owner of your house, as your partner or spouse may jointly own the property. If you are intending to remortgage then you will need your co-owner's consent to do so.

As with using your home for security on a loan, this has to be an option that must be carefully considered, in case your business incurs any financial difficulties.

Borrowing against an insurance policy

This has to be an investment-type policy that has been accumulating for a few years and is not linked to your mortgage. Loans taken against an insurance policy usually tend to be for 3 to 5 years or over.

Problems with loans

It may be possible for you to pay off a loan early for some reason. If you wish to do so, check that there is not a financial penalty involved in early payment. Banks are keen to loan money, and customers may well be in a position to negotiate the terms of the deal. You may wish not to have loans or all your policies with one agency, e.g. the bank. If there are financial problems, the bank will be very quick to seize your assets.

Surrendering a life policy

Only certain policies can be surrendered. These are usually the investment-type policies, which pay bonuses at intervals and add up to a reasonable sum once the policy has finished.

A life policy usually takes a few years to build up to a point at which it has a surrender value. Therefore, the more recent the policy, the less money you will be able to get out of it. If you choose to cash it in too early, you may get back less money than you have paid in premiums.

If the policy has matured sufficiently, you will get out more than you paid in but you will lose out on the final bonus. It may, therefore, be better to keep your policy intact and use it as security against a loan.

Special loans, grants and bursaries

Finding out what is available requires research and persistence. This type of information is available at libraries; librarians have up-to-date information about these grants on their online databases. The Internet is also a valuable resource.

There are many grants available, but they may alter fairly rapidly.

- The DTI and Business Link websites (see p. 249) are useful gateways to learning about grants.
- Information about local enterprise agencies (LEAs) and local enterprise companies (LECs) is available through the Scottish Enterprise website (see p. 249).

The Prince's Trust

This can help unemployed young people aged between 18 and 30 to start their own businesses by providing not only financial assistance and marketing opportunities, but also an ongoing mentoring system to monitor their progress. There is also a free legal helpline, which is available 24 hours a day, 7 days a week, to any business currently supported by The Prince's Trust.

Providing applicants have a viable business idea and are able to convince the trust of their initiative and commitment, they will be considered. They must also be able to prove that they have not been able to obtain funding from any other source, for example a bank loan.

The loan is not large but can be helpful in getting your business off the ground, and you will not have to provide security to get it. You will be expected to produce a business plan. There is, however, a large team of volunteers with extensive business experience who will be able to assist you with producing an appropriate plan.

Highlands and Islands Enterprise

It may be worth looking at this, although they are particularly interested in ventures that involve production, tourism, and information technology.

Conclusion

There are a large number of ways to finance your business. Before choosing one you must consider several factors:

- *Do you need a loan?* In many circumstances complementary therapists are able, given a little thought, to start quite simply without compromising professionalism. This may require you to be a part-time therapist for a while until you are busy enough to work full time in your chosen field.
- *Have you thoroughly worked through all the stages that lead up to producing a business plan and the finances associated with it?* Cost calculations and marketing should have all been thoroughly researched and your figures checked by someone who is experienced in these matters. At the end of the day if the figures you produce make no sense, the lender will not even start to contemplate giving you a loan.
- *Have you got a support network in place?* This may range from someone who has business experience to someone who is able to support you emotionally and make your life easier while you start up. Taking on a loan can initially be very stressful if you have never run your own business before.
- *Do you have the cooperation of your family, particularly spouse or partner, if you are going to put the finances at risk?* If this is likely to become a source of strain to the relationship, then it may be necessary to think again about how you fund your business.

Useful websites

Australia

http://www.business.gov.au/Business+Entry+Point/Business+Topics/Grants+assistance/

Australian Government
Business website – grants and funding. Links to different governmental areas.

Canada

Many websites are bilingual.

http://bsa.cbsc.org/gol/bsa/site.nsf/en/index.html

Canadian government's start-up assistant
This covers all the territories. Provides useful information on finding finance.

New Zealand

Governmental websites are bilingual.

http://www.biz.org.nz/public/Section.aspx?SectionID=46&FromSectionID=38

Business Information Zone
Grants and financial assistance.

UK

http://www.businesslink.gov.uk/

Business Link

http://www.dti.gov.uk/

Department of Trade and Industry

http://www.hie.co.uk/

Highlands and Islands Enterprise

http://www.princes-trust.org.uk/

The Prince's Trust

http://www.scottish-enterprise.com/sedotcom_home/about_se/local_enterprise_companies.htm

Scottish Enterprise

USA

http://www.business.gov/

Business.gov

http://www.firstgov.gov/

United States Government

http://www.sba.gov/

United States Small Business Administration

Part 4

Procedure

Clinic procedure 19

Chapter contents

Every clinic no matter how big or small has to have some sort of procedure for its everyday running. On a larger scale the clinic may be run by a practice manager, but as you are unlikely to be able to afford such a useful member of staff immediately, unless you have a willing relative or friend who will perform the task, this job will be down to you.

Many colleges produce a clinic handbook, which can be a very useful document and should not be discarded after qualifying. Adapt it for your own practice procedures and use it as a reference.

Being organized

Organization is not only the mark of a competent practitioner, but of an administrator as well. Disorganization will lead to loss of documentation and financial difficulties through mismanagement.

Disorganization usually comes through an unwillingness to do something and using procrastination to temporarily push the task to one side. Some jobs are more important than others and there does need to be a certain amount of prioritization, but a task initially pushed to the back of the queue will need to be dealt with at some point or it will come back to haunt you.

When you are starting out, with the best will in the world, it is not always possible to book all your patients right next to each other and you will have gaps. If you are likely to be working in the day to support your fledgling clinic and then in the evening or weekends with not much spare time available, then work out clinic procedure ahead of time. If you have a system in place, organization is so much easier.

Organization can be as simple as putting stationery in a specific location, so that you always know where to find it.

General paperwork

Paperwork is probably the area where the most disorganization occurs. This is because it is boring and not the reason why you studied so hard for several years to become qualified in your particular therapy.

If you are not an organized person, then start simply.

Bills. Pay them straight away and put the invoice, with the date and means of payment recorded on it, immediately into a file. If you want to leave payment to a certain date, then put these invoices in a file or folder in a special place where you routinely check on them. Having this routine in place will mean you can deal with them before the payment deadline is reached.

Prioritize paperwork. Quickly read through new paperwork, be it bills or letters, and put a priority on it immediately. If you cannot deal with it at once then it should be filed in order with a time limit on it that should not be exceeded.

Accounts. Once you have paid for something, enter it in your ledger. It is always best to do everything as soon as possible. Once the task is finished you will then be able to give your full attention to the next one. There is nothing more demotivating than a pile of unattended invoices. Many unpaid bills have been a result of loss of documentation rather than lack of money in the bank.

Forming good habits is important. Studies have shown that if you perform a task on a regular basis for 28 days, you become patterned and the task becomes a routine. This works for good as well as bad habits.

Being organized does give a great sense of well-being, since you will know exactly which tasks need attending to and which you have completed.

Mail

Junk mail. Throw this out as soon as it arrives or it will pile up.

General mail. When you become busy it may be worth considering a mail book, particularly if someone else, such as your receptionist, is preparing and posting the mail. This will tell you what has come in and gone out and on what date.

Evidence of posting. For extra assurance that something has been posted, a certificate of posting can be obtained from the post office.

Recorded delivery. If it is important that documents such as case histories and X-rays are signed for at the other end you can send post by recorded delivery and receipts can be clipped to the mail book, or into your bank pay-in book if the money you have used has come out of your takings.

Taking calls

Although high-quality treatment is a mainstay of your clinic, you need to get the patients in to treat them. The way a call is dealt with is vital to the success of your clinic. If it is handled badly then potential patients will lose confidence in you before they get anywhere near the clinic, so it is worth having a routine for answering the phone in an efficient and informative manner.

If you do not feel spontaneous on the phone, write down useful phrases or a checklist of what you need to go through with a patient. You will probably need this anyway if you rent a room and use a communal receptionist or if you get your own receptionist.

The basic details you need are:

- *The patient's name and contact number.* This enables you to ring patients who do not attend for any reason or if you have to change an appointment. Some practitioners also take the patient's address before the first visit because they need to send out information beforehand or need forms filling in, or simply because they charge for non-attendance of the first consultation.
- *Your charges.* It can be awkward if patients are not aware of these and find after the treatment that the cost is more than they expected. So let them know before they come to see you.
- *Directions.* If you are not local to the area, take the time to go out onto the major routes to make a note of landmarks and all the quirks of the route (such as one-way streets) to help steer people in. If people have

trouble finding you they may give up. Providing your postcode is useful now the use of satellite navigation is becoming more common. If you have a website, make use of a clear location map. Even if you do not have a website, advertising with an online company such as Yell.com will result in your being linked to a location-finding service.

- *Be able to give a clear, but concise description of exactly what it is you do and what you treat.* Many people may not know or understand your particular therapy and are ringing up for an explanation. Having an explanation ready and being able to quickly and concisely answer their questions will display your professionalism and make them confident of your abilities.
- *What do you do if it is not clear to either you or the patient whether your treatment is applicable?* Many clinics offer a short appointment for which no charge is made. This enables the practitioner and the patient to meet face to face and for the practitioner to assess whether the treatment is appropriate, but at that stage a diagnosis should not be given.

  Since this is not a consultation, great care should be taken to make it clear that the appointment is only an evaluation. Some professional bodies strongly suggest that the practitioner keeps a record of the meeting along with consent for the evaluation.
- *Be helpful.* If your treatment is not appropriate or you cannot accommodate the patient at that time, explain why and suggest a suitable alternative. This will ensure that the patient is treated by someone who is both competent and qualified. If that patient has a different problem in the future you may be the first one to be called.

Answering calls while treating

It is not a good idea to answer a call while you are treating a patient. The patient is entitled to your complete attention, and taking calls while a patient is with you can detract from the treatment or may result in your having a conversation that is not appropriate for someone else to hear.

If you are expecting a call that is important and cannot be avoided, as may be the case where, for example, you are trying to have a vital conversation with a colleague who has the same problem of availability as you, explain to the patient at the start of the treatment. Try to be brief and if possible leave the room.

If for any other reason you do have to take a call during treatment, keep the conversation short, probably taking the details of the caller's name and telephone number so you can ring back at a more convenient time.

Using an answering machine

Many practitioners cannot afford the luxury of a receptionist when they first start out, so an answering machine is the next best thing.

Unfortunately, many people tend to put the phone down the minute they hear an answering machine, but some do wait to hear what is said before making a decision. This is where what you put on the machine can make the difference between a message being left for you and losing a potential patient.

- *Use as much variation in tone as possible.* This may sound ridiculous while you are speaking, but on playback your voice should appear warm and inviting. Try it several times with different tones of voice and placing your emphasis in different places. You could also try playing the sample messages to your friends to see which sounds the best to them. Finally, ring up your answering machine with the message on it to hear exactly what a patient will be hearing.
- *Endeavour to give the impression that you will ring back as quickly as possible.* Let callers know the approximate time by which you will return their call. For example, you may say that you are treating a patient and this means you will ring back as soon as you are free. If you have to be out of the clinic or cannot take a call for a period of time, tell the caller when you will be in a position to return the call; for example, if you are having a lunch break, treating patients or have closed for the weekend. This lets potential patients know you are there and that they are not just listening to a standard message that is always left on the answering machine regardless of time or day.

Mobile phones

For a practitioner just starting up a mobile phone is an essential item. Not only are you able to divert calls to your mobile, but you will also be able to put your own specific message onto voicemail, and most of the time (unless the caller's number has been withheld) see who has rung you.

The flexibility of this system will mean that you can go out during the day to attend to jobs that need be done, and does not mean you have to sit in your clinic waiting for calls.

If you do work from someone else's property, where you might not have a receptionist or may not be allowed to the use the phone, you will still be able to have your own dedicated clinic phone by diverting calls to your mobile.

Although mobile calls are more expensive than a landline and you pick up the cost of the mobile call if it is put through a divert system, it is still cheaper and less involved than hiring a receptionist.

If possible, always have a landline number for your clinic phone, since mobile numbers do not give a sense of permanence to prospective patients. Once you are treating a patient, the mobile number allows the patient to maintain contact with you even when you are not in the clinic. It is a system that is usually rarely used, but knowing you are available at these times is reassuring to the patient.

Taking bookings

Receptionists

A good receptionist is invaluable and a bad one is a disaster since bad receptionists are able to lose potential patients before they even make an appointment.

Your receptionist is the patients' first port of call. If he is good at the job, patients will be completely at ease with him and will not be concerned that they are not speaking directly to a practitioner.

A good receptionist should be someone who is:

- *Conversant with your therapy.* Take time to explain what it is you do. You cannot expect your receptionist to be an expert, but your professional body should supply leaflets that describe what the patient can expect in the way of treatment. If the receptionist is unsure of whether your treatment is appropriate after a conversation with a prospective patient, he could take the phone number and say you will ring the person back, or offer a screening consultation to see if the therapy you offer is suitable for the condition.
- *A good conversationalist,* but someone who knows when to give the patient space.
- *Able to handle people,* enabling the most nervous of patients to be relaxed the minute they walk through the door.
- *Discrete and respectful of confidentiality.* The receptionist will handle patient files and therefore will have access to them, particularly if you have a database, which needs to be kept up to date.
- *Self-motivated.* Receptionists should be able to perform tasks and organize themselves without needing to be constantly directed. These days a receptionist not only needs to have good telephone skills, but some knowledge of how to use a computer such as for typing letters and entering details onto a database.
- *Good at basic administration.* There is always some paperwork with a busy clinic, and as many clinics are now expected to self-audit, the receptionist may be responsible for organizing this.
- *Competent with basic arithmetic,* as he will be handling money.
- *Honest.* Your receptionist will be handling a great deal of cash when you become busy. When you hire someone, do take time to check his references, a task often overlooked by practitioners who are too embarrassed or to preoccupied to do this.

Do bear in mind the running cost and legal complexities of employing someone, when you first establish your clinic.

Working from a multidisciplinary clinic that takes bookings for you

Keep one clinic diary at that particular clinic if someone else is taking the bookings. There is nothing to stop you having your own book, but it must be made very clear who is responsible for bookings so you do not end up double booked or worse having a patient booked in you do not know about. If the clinic you work at makes the bookings, then have a system where the patient list is checked with you before they close on the day before you come in to see patients.

Alternatives to a receptionist

Wherever possible have someone to answer the phone for you, even if that person is a relative. As long as people have a good telephone manner, a reasonable idea of what you can do, and have been adequately briefed, they can book patients in.

If they are not sure whether your particular therapy can help, they should take the potential patient's telephone number and assure the patient that you will ring them back. The call should be returned as quickly as possible.

Computers in the clinic

Possessing a computer is not necessary when first starting out, although many households do have one.

Accounts and appointments can be easily entered into ledgers and appointments books.

There are advantages to computerization, particularly with the sophistication of hand-held computers, which can be synchronized with the main clinic computer. The appointments can be quickly downloaded and uploaded so you always have a running account of the clinic day.

It is vital, however, to back up the information on the computer, as electronic storage devices can so easily crash and lose information.

Clinical paperwork

Case history forms

It goes without saying that you must have some type of case history form. Good, clear records are essential. They are vital for effective patient management, since they track the patient's progress. In these days of increasing litigation a clear record can prove to be very useful.

You will, at some point, need to go on holiday and whoever acts as your locum or covers for you will be able to give a seamless treatment.

Case history forms can now be produced to a high quality on a computer. Once your template is stored, the form can be printed out when required.

You may wish the patient to fill in the patient case history form in the waiting room. This may be as little as name and address and doctor or can amount to a complete medical questionnaire, which you then elaborate on.

Certainly some professional bodies now state that, as a matter of course before treatment, the patient should read an information sheet on what to expect, as part of the process of being adequately informed. As most professional bodies produce a more than adequate leaflet, you should not need to produce your own.

The case history form will then not only contain the patient's details, but also the patient's signature for consent. In some cases, practitioners have required a patient signature for three separate items.

- To indicate the patient has read and understood the contents of the information leaflet
- Consent for examination
- Consent for treatment.

Certainly, consent for treatment is vital.

Ask patients to come in early for their initial consultation, so that they have opportunity to read the leaflet and fill in any necessary forms.

Transferring a patient to another practitioner

It is inevitable that patients will move away or need to see another practitioner. If this is the case and they are with you for their last visit, try to arrange their next appointment for them if they require ongoing treatment.

It is much more professional to arrange the appointment directly from your clinic, and arrange for the patient's notes to be transferred. If it is more expedient for patients to take a copy of their own notes and you have photocopying facilities to hand, then the process is simplified as patients can be given a copy of their notes to take with them, providing they sign for them.

It can be helpful to keep a logbook for all the occasions notes are copied and sent to other clinics. This way you will have an accurate record of what confidential documents have left the clinic. The details included may be:

- *Date.*
- *Name of patient.*
- *Authorization of patient.* Where this is being held.
- *Signature of person taking copy.* If it has been taken by hand.
- *Signature of person overseeing the handover.* This may be the practitioner or another nominated person.

- *X-rays associated with the file.* These are generally sent, so note needs to be made of how they were transferred. They should be sent by recorded delivery.
- *Return of X-rays.* X-rays may be sent to a consultant, then returned. This will tell you if the X-rays are still absent from the clinic.
- *Date X-rays returned.*

Otherwise the patient's signature on the original notes or the consent form for transferring the notes should be in the patient file.

If a patient is transferring to another clinic and that clinic rings to request the notes, it is a good idea to ask for written authorization from the patient.

Some clinics have reciprocal arrangements where verbal permission from the patient is adequate for copies or X-rays to be sent, but a record should still be kept.

Keeping track of records is important. It is not unknown for solicitors to ask for records going back as far as 6 years.

Certificates for illness

Many complementary therapists can now sign a certificate to show that a patient has good reason to be off work. Patients should, however, sign themselves off in the first week, but after that they will require some official notification.

If you do use the certificate the key points to note are:

- *If you feel that the patient is going to require an inordinately long period off work, then it is probably better that the GP is informed and takes responsibility for this task.* General practitioners do not appreciate being informed of a condition that is not resolving, several weeks after treatment has commenced.
- *The diagnosis given should be precise.* For example, putting 'back pain' is not adequate.
- *It is a good idea to have a clinic stamp for the box requiring details of the practitioner's qualifications, name and address.* This space can be very small, so it is also a good idea when constructing your clinic stamp for more general items, such as leaflets, to ensure it fits everything you are likely to stamp.

Blood donor certificate

If you pierce the skin during the course of treatment, for example if you are an acupuncturist or a chiropractor qualified to perform dry needling, your professional body should have made arrangements for you to issue blood donor certificates to confirm that your patients are being treated by a competent and professionally trained practitioner.

If patients are unable to present one of these certificates each year, they will not be able to give blood.

Cancellations

Your position on cancellation can be posted on the clinic notice board and/or stated on a small notice on your business card.

It is useful to say that if patients have to cancel, they should give you 24 hours notice or they will have to pay a cancellation fee.

Music

You may play music in your reception area to improve the ambiance or, in cases where there is only a door between you and reception, to ensure confidentiality. You may also play music in the room for patient relaxation, for example while treating using massage.

If this is the case then you must be aware that this constitutes a 'public performance', even if you use the radio, and technically you should register with the Performing Rights Society (website, p. 268). There is an annual fee.

You can buy tapes or CDs or can download music from the Royalty Free Music website (see p. 268). For this you pay a one-off payment that allows you to use the music whenever you want.

Security

Property

Insurance companies will not pay out for theft if the property owner has not made suitable arrangements for security of equipment or personal property.

If you lock the entrance door between treatments, then install a doorbell so you can go to let the patient in.

If the entrance door to your clinic is unlocked while you are with a patient, then either a receptionist should be there or you need an alarm on the door that makes a noise when someone comes in. These systems usually come in a kit and are easily fitted since they can be powered by a battery. Many of these systems can be linked to the general alarm system.

It is advisable if you work in a multi-practitioner clinic practice and you have a room that can be locked, to do so every time you leave the room. It is very easy in a large and busy clinic for an intruder to enter with a view to opportunist theft.

If you have staff, then you should supply some means of securing personal items such as handbags, since these are attractive to thieves and easy to remove.

Working from home poses another problem since theft has a much more personal aspect to it. Do check with your insurance policy as to the coverage you are likely to receive and whether you are required to take extra measures such as putting locks on your internal doors.

It may be advisable to find some way to isolate the clinic area from the rest of the house if it has a separate entrance. Alternatively, lock all the rooms in the house if they are not being used. Normally patients should not be out of your sight so this should not be an issue.

Generally it is better to only allow access to the house under your control and not leave the outside doors open unless there is someone there to supervise entry.

During a holiday period, a keyholder must be available to deal with any problems such as a break-in or alarm system problems.

Equipment

This includes acupuncture needles and herbs, which should be secured from general access if they are stored outside the treatment room. This is not so much to guard against theft as for the safety of the general public who will enter your premises. Care should also be taken of equipment in your treatment room if patients are present, particularly if they have children with them.

Used needles should be deposited in a sharps box along with any material used to swab spots of blood. There are many firms now that provide reasonable services without a contract. A moderate fee of £8–10 will cover delivery of a bucket and a replacement on removal of the old bucket.

Lasers should have a key which can be removed. If it is likely that you will have a child in the room with you when you are treating the parent, the laser will not be used anyway, so remove the key. If you work in a multi-practitioner clinic and the room cannot be locked, remove the key into your safekeeping every time you leave.

Personal

Personal security is always a risk, and although it does not appear to have been a big issue in the profession so far, it is worth considering.

Working from home

Working from home poses the biggest problem, as you may be on your own. If you are unsure, tell patients you will ring them back when you are free. This tends to deter anyone who is not genuine. Usually the conversations you have had with your potential patients will tell you a great deal about the type of people they are.

No matter how professionally you present yourself there may be times where a patient can misread the signals you give off.

Key aspects to maintaining personal safety are:

- *Ensure you have the appropriate back-up in case trouble arises.*
- *Know what to do if trouble does arise.*

- *Try to ensure that any enquiry for your services is genuine and that you and your prospective patient know what to expect from the treatment.*
- *Work from reputable premises.*

Domiciliary visits

Many practitioners still do domiciliary visits, and the list above on maintaining personal security applies, together with the following:

- *Word-of-mouth referrals are usually the safest type of booking.* On the principle that like attracts like, you should have a good idea of what type of person you are going to visit.
- *Check out the area you are going to before you make the visit* or at least see if someone you know well can tell you about it.
- *Take a companion with you on your first house call to an unknown patient.*
- *If you have the slightest doubt, refuse to take the patient.*
- *If you are a woman who is going on a house call to a man, is another woman going to be present, and the reverse if you are a male practitioner?*
- *Leave a schedule with someone who will expect you to ring at set times.*
- *Set up the treatment space so that you are between the patient and the door.*

Time spent with patients

It is important to keep to time, whenever possible. The time needed can vary from one profession to another and, within the profession, between individuals.

If you do have a clock in your room, try to place it where you are aware of it but your patient is not. The clock should also be quiet, as a loud relentless tick becomes very obtrusive after a time.

No matter how limited your time, do not give the impression to the patient that you are rushed. If you do have a tendency to run behind, leave catch-up gaps.

If you are running very late, give the waiting patients an idea of the delay, in case they have a tight schedule. Make them as comfortable as possible, with a drink of tea or coffee, and make sure you have newspapers or interesting and up-to-date magazines for them to read. Most people do not mind waiting if they are occupied.

Maintaining décor

As your clinic gets busier, it is likely to incur some wear. General decoration will need to be done every few years, but areas that get particularly marked will need to be dealt with more frequently.

Occasionally take time to sit or lie in the patient's position, as this will enable you to see the clinic from the patients' perspective. Are there any spiders' webs hanging from the light fittings, or cracks in the ceiling? It is amazing what patients focus on if they are in one position for any length of time.

Conclusion

It is a good idea to develop a system of clinic procedure right from the start. Obviously this will need to be adapted as time goes on, but the basic mechanics of what does work will not change.

Establishing a routine early on means that, as the clinic becomes busier, you will have no problems keeping on top of all the little tasks, which if not done will as a whole become overwhelming.

Many of the everyday activities you will engage in with your clinic will ultimately require some strategy to allow you to cope with the myriad of tasks, and Chapter 21 enlarges on some strategies to help you cope with your everyday routine if it seems somewhat hectic.

Most importantly, have an eye for details and constantly check them, because 'the devil is in the details', and if you do not pay attention to them, they will soon make themselves known.

Useful websites

Australia

http://www.apra.com.au/

Australian Performing Rights Association

Canada

Many websites are bilingual.

http://www.socan.ca/music/royalty.html

Socan
Canadian performing rights, composers, lyricists, songwriters, publishers, licence.

New Zealand

Governmental websites are bilingual.

http://www.apra.co.nz/licences.htm

Australian Performing Rights Association

http://www.rianz.org.nz/rianz/PPNZ.asp

Phonographic Performances New Zealand
You will need both licences. For further information:

http://www.biz.org.nz/public/content.aspx?sectionid=36&contentid=1863

Business Information Zone
Public performance licence information.

UK

http://www.prs.co.uk/

Performing Rights Society

http://www.royaltyfreemusic.com

Royalty Free Music

USA

http://www.ascap.com/index.html

American Society of Composers, Authors and Publishers

Working with the conventional medical profession

20

Chapter contents

The reception a complementary practitioner receives from the conventional medical profession can vary greatly. There is currently a general awareness of the complementary therapies engendered by the various professional bodies, who are working hard to provide accurate information and relevant research to further their cause.

It is therefore entirely appropriate for an individual practitioner to build bridges by working to increase the depth of knowledge possessed by the conventional medical profession about complementary therapy. To do this is to be able to dispel harmful myths and engender understanding, for the benefit of the patient.

Initial contacts

There are usually two main ways in which your local surgeries will become aware of your presence:

- Patient reports.
- Direct contact.

Patient reports

Traditionally, this has been the usual way that complementary practitioners have had of making their presence known.

Advantages

- *It is a good way to develop trust between you and the conventional profession.* If enough patients report back then your reputation builds.
- *It is likely to result in a lasting relationship.* Once trust has been established, then it is very likely you will be mentioned to patients if the type of treatment you give is appropriate.

Disadvantages

- *This method of referral can take a long time.* It will take time for your reputation to build, and although practitioners may have become aware of your presence they still do not know you personally, so referral can be erratic.
- *Patient dissatisfaction.* If patients have been dissatisfied with your treatment or feel they have been made worse by it, they will be as, or more, voluble with criticism than they would have been in praising you.

Direct contact

Since relying on patient word of mouth can be slow and erratic, contacting the orthodox practitioners who have involvement with your patient is a good idea. Anyone responds more favourable to someone they have had the opportunity to meet face to face to discuss the therapy that is on offer.

Contact can occur in two ways: by a practitioner's letter, or by self-introduction.

A practitioner's letter

You may need to make the GP aware of a patient's condition, because it is either inappropriate to treat the patient or important for the GP to know you are seeing the patient, who may require diagnostic tests that cannot be performed by you, e.g. blood tests or X-rays.

This is also the way you are likely to contact a specialist, if the patient you are seeing is either due to go to an initial consultation or is currently seeing a consultant and visiting you with the consultant's knowledge.

Self-introduction

Who Do You Contact? Practice managers are usually the best point of first contact. Find out the manager's name before you contact a practice, so you are able to ask for him by name.

Practice managers send general letters around the internal mail system if they feel they are of relevance, so that all the staff will get a chance to see them. Ring first to get a feel for the reception you are likely to receive. Then if the contact is positive you will be able to send your details and possibly arrange a talk if there is interest.

This is where having professionally printed headed notepaper and business cards will give a good impression. If you do not have your own practice leaflet then use the one produced by your professional body, making sure it is stamped with your name and address. Enclose your CV if it is relevant or at least a short résumé. Relevant statistics and research are useful even if the surgery has already received a general information package.

Liaising with hospitals

Contact with your local hospital is normally in the form of a practitioner letter. If your patient is going to see a consultant in the outpatient department of a hospital then give your letter directly to the patient. This ensures that it gets directly to the consultant. If the consultant is being seen privately then the letter can be posted, or taken by the patient.

Once members of a conventional medical profession start a working relationship with a complementary therapist, which may vary from a verbal suggestion that a patient should see you to an actual referral letter, usually for a medical healthcare insurance company, they continue to refer to you since they feel confident in your abilities. The building of trust is one of the most important factors in this type of referral.

Content of letters

Letters need to be brief and, if possible, printed on A5 paper, which fits more easily into the patient record wallets. Surgeries are working towards a paperless system, so although hard copies will be retained, correspondence is now scanned by most surgeries so it can be computerized. For this reason the letter should be written or typed onto paper so that it can be easily legible when it is scanned.

The important points for a letter are:

- *Keep it brief*, but make sure it contains all the relevant points.
- *Doctor's or consultant's name and address.* Usually the full address of doctors (this can be found from the NHS website (see p. 275) where there is a search engine for all the doctors' surgeries in the UK).
- *Patient's name, address, date of birth.* Make sure you use the patient's actual first name and not a nickname, because that is how it will be logged in.
- *Avoid specialized non-medical terms.* For example, most doctors will not understand Chinese medical terms.
- *Your diagnosis*, if you are able to give one, or at least an indication of what signs or symptoms the patient is displaying that make you want another opinion.

- *What treatment you are giving the patient.*
- *What you would like the GP to do.* If you do not know the practitioner well or do not feel qualified to make this direction, then say that you have found certain signs which indicate something that needs further investigation and have sent the patient to seek advice from the GP regarding this matter.

If you do not have a computer and need to write a letter while a patient is with you so that she can take it with her, a clear handwritten letter is perfectly acceptable. Do photocopy it if you can or make a note of what you have said.

Giving talks

The conventional medical profession is now becoming more aware that the complementary field has something to offer, and does try to arrange talks to their medical staff for continuing professional development (CPD), post-graduate training for registrars and even talks for medical students. Although you may end up talking to a large group of doctors and nurses who may or may not continue to work in the area, it is likely that you will be remembered when they need a therapist.

It is possible to arrange a talk yourself. This can be given at your clinic, the surgery or another meeting place. Do bear in mind that doctors have a responsibility to people who cannot wait to see them and as a consequence you may end up with fewer people than you started with at the beginning of your talk, if they are called out.

Do consider the location carefully. For example, bringing doctors into your premises does allow them to see exactly how you work, but it might be difficult for them to get there if they are on call. Therefore, holding the talk at their place of work and where they feel comfortable might ensure that members of your audience can return after they have dealt with a situation that requires their attention.

Because GPs are so short of time, an incentive, such as refreshments or the ability to count the event towards their CPD, is a good idea. Contact the local postgraduate educational facility to get details of how to register yourself as a Continuing Professional Development provider. Then, every time GPs attend one of your talks, they will be able to claim CPD points.

Individual appointments

These are very difficult to get unless the GP is very interested in what you have to offer. GPs do have a limited time in the day available for such appointments, when they will see such people as drugs representatives, but they may be booked as far as 6 months ahead or more.

Points to bear in mind when talking to the conventional medical profession

- *Be professional.* Dressing smartly does help create a good impression.
- *Be enthusiastic.* As with any business, your enthusiasm will go a long way to further your cause.
- *Be clear about what your treatment can do to help patients.* Largely, the conventional medical profession will want to know what you can treat, how long it might take and how much it costs.
- *Be prepared to back up your claims regarding treatment.* It is not enough to say that your particular treatment has been in use a long time. Do not forget that in referring patients to you, GPs still have the responsibility of being the primary carer for that patient, so they have to be sure that the referral is made on substantial grounds.
- *Do not criticize another practitioner.* If you feel strongly about the inadequacy of another complementary practitioner, keep it to yourself. Concentrate instead on the standards upheld by your professional body and the educational establishment you graduated from.
- *State the requirements made by professional bodies.* Many orthodox practitioners have no idea of the standards that have to be achieved by many of the complementary professions, or that they have codes of ethics and safe practice and audit requirements.

How funding works

It is possible to treat patients with special governmental, European or National Health Service funding; however, it is difficult to obtain. Unless the new practitioner is extremely ambitious and has previous experience of dealing with this type of bureaucracy, then it is best left alone until more clinical experience is gained.

There are several reasons for this:

- *Clinical proficiency is a priority.* If you are occupied with form filling, making calls and having meetings you will not be able to embark on probably the most important part of your career, acquiring polished clinical skills.
- *It is essential to establish a steady patient base.* You need to be in a position to pay off your debts or at least start working full time in your clinic as quickly as possible. NHS funding is done on a contractual basis and can therefore be cut or entirely removed from year to year. Other funds may only last for a certain period of time. The private sector is still the most reliable source of income. You must remain economically viable.
- *There is substantial paperwork involved.* This will require statistics associated with your clinic, so your clinic needs to have some history.

Clinical audits and precise accounting are also very important. If you are starting from scratch then you will have to do extensive research, probably lasting months, to justify your cause (read about the Impact project in Nottingham (website, p. 274) to get insight into this).

- *You may not get paid the going rate.* Do not forget that you should be properly compensated for your expertise. General prices are always rising, so your charges will also need to do so, to match. If you are on a contract, you will be required to work at the price agreed in your contract regardless of any other change.

Conclusion

Once you have won their trust, members of the conventional medical profession can become very enthusiastic champions of complementary medicine.

Considering the moves afoot to look at a health service where integration is an everyday occurrence, this situation can only improve.

Whatever your reasons for liaising with conventional medicine, creating a healthy interface can only result in ensuring the best quality of care for your patients.

Useful websites

http://www.fihealth.org.uk/

Prince of Wales Foundation for Integrated Health
This site has useful information on the integration of complementary medicine and conventional medicine. The document 'A Healthy Partnership: Integrating Complementary Healthcare Into Primary Care' is particularly useful.

http://www.impact-imp.co.uk

Nottingham Impact Project
This website is useful for the links and downloads, offering an insight into obtaining grant money for a specific community to enable integrated healthcare. It also offers an analysis of the success of the project.

http://www.integratedhealth.org.uk

Somerset Trust for Integrated Healthcare
Complementary therapy in general practice. This website presents findings from the work of the Glastonbury Health Centre Complementary Medicine Service.

http://www.kingsfund.org.uk/index.html

The King's Fund

This is an independent charitable foundation working for better health, especially in London. There is a useful download on 'Clinical Governance for Complementary and Alternative Medicine in Primary Healthcare'.

http://www.nhs.uk/

National Health Service

21 Strategies for coping with the demands on you while you are developing your clinic

Chapter contents

You are now at the stage where your own clinic is no longer a project in the future, but a reality. You have only treated a few patients, but are learning not only about treatment, but also what does and does not work for you in the general running of the clinic.

It is unusual for practitioners to be able to immediately devote full-time attention to a new practice without the need to supplement their income in some way. Even if you do not need to take out a loan or overdraft, you should have put a business plan together, or at the very least have a very clear picture of how much money you need to generate a month to live on and how much is available for general expenditure. As you build up your clinic you should see the income grow and reach a point where it is possible to become a full-time practitioner.

Until this time, however, you are having a physically and mentally demanding time, where you are torn between the desire to attend to your new venture, and the need to earn money to fulfil your everyday financial demands. You will also experience a fluctuation of your patient load throughout the year because of events such as public holidays, which can interfere with your calculations. You will not be on your own in this, and many very successful practitioners will relate similar stories.

Successful businesspeople develop the skills to deal with these situations so that they can cope with the demands made on them when they are working flat out and use the quieter periods as opportunities to reappraise and move the business forward.

There will probably be two main categories of new practitioners:

- Those who are able to devote a full day, or at least half a day, once or a few times a week to their own enterprise.
- Those who initially will have to work very unsociable hours to fit around a nine-to-five job.

So how do you go about ensuring you remain positive within a situation that might be less than ideal?

I never seem to have enough time

One of the major concerns of new practitioners, or those attempting to go full time, is the apparent lack of hours in the day and the loss of the personal space they previously enjoyed.

First of all it is important to view this in perspective and realize that this should be a very short period in relation to the rest of your working life. Then view your day from the point of view of organization and ask yourself whether you are using the time you do have to devote to your new clinic as effectively as possible. There will be certain administrative needs around seeing patients and the need to ensure that your name is going out positively into the community in order to build up business, but there should also be a certain amount of time outside your place of work for you and your family.

So how do you reconcile your work as a business owner, practitioner and private individual?

There are a few simple things that can be done before getting into detailed analysis:

- *Try to keep everything tidy.* If you use something put it away in the same place again, so you do not waste time trying to locate it.
- *Deal with your paperwork constructively.* This has been dealt with in more detail in the chapter on clinic procedure (Ch. 19). A great deal of time can be saved if you are not wading through large and confusing amounts of paperwork because items are in no particular order.
- *Delegate when you can.* For example, is it possible to get someone to do the banking for you, or can someone deal with booking patients and taking the money?

Time management

The expression 'Time is money' can be very true for a busy practitioner. The time you might spend on a non-productive activity could have been time spent seeing a patient. It is possible to think about spending time, as you would think about money. You have already gone through the process of looking at finances, and your approach to the utilization of time could be very similar.

Time management, however, is not purely about chopping your day into 10- or 20-minute time slots, but also about appreciating how much time needs to be allocated to a particular task, along with a sense of prioritization.

There is no shortage of books readily available on the subject of time management. These are a few of the principles to use when starting out:

- *Make lists.* Writing tasks down means that they become visible and therefore less easy to push to one side. A written list also makes it easier to see what needs to do be done and what you have done. Prioritize tasks, and set deadlines for each of them. For example, you may have to prioritize paying bills over networking with other professionals, since you have reached the deadline where they have to be paid. This process, however, may only take a short period of time, so it will be possible to schedule a meeting with a colleague just after it.
- *Keep your lists in a visible place.* This means you will not forget them.
- *Prioritize.* Prioritization does help to narrow your focus. By prioritizing your tasks you will be able to focus on a limited number of tasks in a set period and give them your full attention. You can allocate tasks daily, weekly or monthly.
- *Dedicate certain periods of time to certain activities.* For example, use specific times for phone calls. You can let your patients know when you will be available, or leave a message for anyone ringing in. Alternatively, use your catch-up gap.
- *Keep a log of activities.* If you cannot understand why you never seem to have enough time to complete tasks, keep a log of your activities and be as honest as possible. Although this appears to be another job to add to your growing list, it can be done quickly during the course of the day. The results may surprise you. When you finally start working full time for yourself, then awareness of non-constructive time-filling activities will allow you to use your day effectively and enable you to maintain a positive mental attitude.
- *Do allocate some down time during the day.* There are times in a busy schedule where it is important to have some respite, and regular breaks are something you must include in your daily routine. If you are someone who can feel pressured, then you should alter your appointments to create space. For example, appointments can be spaced further apart or time can be made between patients to incorporate a tea break, both of which will enable you to temporarily unwind. This may make for a slower build-up, but if you are stressed it is more than likely that this will be reflected in the quality of your treatment.
- *Set some time aside where you will not be interrupted.* This may only be 10 minutes, but will be enough to work through something that requires

attention. Turn off the ringers on your telephones and, if working from home, you need to be in your treatment room, having instructed your family not to interrupt you. A few minutes spent this way will be far more productive than an hour of interruptions.

- *Delegate.* Delegation is important for time management and will greatly enhance your efficiency and remove some pressure from your day.
- *Learn to say no.* Some of the most pressured people are those who cannot refuse any job given to them, even if it makes unreasonable demands on their time. You have a duty to yourself, your patients and your family to keep your stress levels down.

Organization of your life using quadrants

The use of quadrants is an interesting one. It is actually only a part of a 'principle-centred' way of managing your life. Using it in isolation does, therefore, have its limitations, but a full explanation is outside the scope of this book. Even so, on its own it can still be of great value to a nascent practitioner. Figure 21.1 represents the activities people engage in and the particular quadrant that is applicable for each activity.

	Urgent	**Not urgent**
Important	I Crises Pressing problems Deadline-driven projects, meetings, preparations	II Preparation Prevention Planning Relationship building
Not important	III Interruptions, some phone calls Some mail, some reports Some meetings Drop-in visitors	IV Trivia Junk mail Some phone calls Time wasters 'Escape' activities

Figure 21.1 Quadrant diagram showing the categories of activities that people engage in. After Covey et al 1999, with permission of Stephen R Covey and Franklin Covey.

Quadrant I is the quadrant of necessity. It represents matters that are *both urgent and important*. This is the area many people operate in as they are fire fighting or crisis managing; for example, paying urgent bills, or performing an urgent repair. If you do not deal with the situations that arise in this area, then they will mount up to a point where you no longer know how to deal with them. If you are permanently in Quadrant I, you will be quickly heading for burnout due to stress.

Quadrant II consists of the activities that are *important but not urgent*. This is the quadrant in which long-term planning takes place and you are anticipating and preventing problems, such as urgent repairs occurring.

Operating in this quadrant, you will be able to hone your skills and learn new ones while engaging in continuous professional development. There is also opportunity to consider your family unit or your personal situation and how to improve it. Recreational activities are included in this quadrant, providing they are beneficial to you and your family's well-being.

This is the quadrant you strive to stay in most of the time.

Quadrant III is *urgent but not important*. Many phone calls and meetings fit into this quadrant. If you spend time in this quadrant then you will be too busy dealing with other people's priorities and expectations to deal with your own situation.

Most people consider they are operating in Quadrant I when they are actually operating in Quadrant III, and it may take a little experience for you to recognize the difference between the two. A way to differentiate between them is to ask yourself if the activity contributed to an important objective or created a benefit. If it did not, then it probably belongs in Quadrant III.

Quadrant IV. People who constantly live in Quadrants I and III very often 'escape' into Quadrant IV for some respite. This category of *not urgent and not important* is where, when you are not busy, your attention may lie.

This is also the quadrant where you engage in 'escape' activities or avoidance behaviour to do anything but the activity you should be applying yourself to. You may end up wasting time with idle chitchat because you think you have nothing to do. This does not include quality time relaxing with your family or friends, which should also be built into your day as an important part of it. Operating in this quadrant is as harmful as spending time in Quadrant I and will lead to your business deteriorating.

New practitioners who find they cannot cope or 'burn out' are probably operating in Quadrants I and III all the time.

Try to recognize the quadrants you are operating in during the week and make a note of them. Referring to these notes should make it relatively easy for you to analyse the different ways in which you have spent your time. The recognition alone that too much has been spent in Quadrants I and III will be the right step in making a change in the way you are living your life.

What do I do with my spare time once I have gone full time?

Once you have, at last, generated enough patients to be able to work for yourself full time, you have to fill the gaps previously occupied by your work elsewhere. Proper utilization of this time is still as vital as it ever was.

If there are gaps between patients during your working day, it is even more vital to use some type of timetable to keep yourself constructively busy, even if it is something personal, for example keeping yourself fit. Keeping yourself fit improves your self-esteem, increases your energy levels and therefore your capacity to think.

Your daily plan will have to contain some flexibility, since new patients or existing patients may want to book in, but a list of tasks will give you things to do and achieve, therefore keeping you feeling positive.

If a problem arises, you will have the time to look at it from every angle. There is usually some way out of a problem, it is just necessary to give it careful consideration.

Ensure that you have got everything right.

What you can do if you cannot leave the clinic

There are plenty of activities to keep you occupied. For example:

- Reviewing patient case history forms.
- Catching up on paperwork.
- Reviewing administrative procedure.
- Re-examining your business plan.
- Looking at methods of patient referral.
- Taking calls.

Reviewing case history forms

Despite the number of student clinics you may have attended during your education, they are never quite the same as treating a patient by yourself in your own clinic without the immediate support of your tutors.

The period before your patient load builds to occupy a full day is one of the most valuable times you will have for learning from your cases. Use every new patient as a learning tool and do background reading. This is merely a continuation of your education and, if you are an effective practitioner, you will never stop learning. This process should be enhanced by any postgraduate courses and CPD requirements.

This type of assessment becomes more difficult as patients start to accumulate in numbers, although all practitioners, no matter how experienced, should reassess their treatments from time to time.

Examining every aspect of the case history form will achieve several goals:

- *To see whether you might have questioned the patient in more detail.* Would you have done anything differently? If so, why? Generally your training will ensure that you have noted everything of importance, but there may be small nuances that an experienced practitioner would have picked up on that may have escaped you at the time. Make a note to go back to whatever it was you feel the need to go over again.
- *To find out more about a patient's medication.* The British National Formulary (BNF) is now available online (see p. 285), providing you register. This is free of charge and allows you to see exactly what the patient's medication is being used for and its side-effects.
- *To consider whether other factors such as past medical and family history or lifestyle are relevant to a patient's condition.*

Picking through cases in this way will enable you to be more precise in your treatment and avoid missing out on important signs and symptoms.

Above all, this is time to revise your education. Look at case history forms of both your successes and those you have struggled with, and see what else you might have done.

All of this work will greatly enhance your abilities as a practitioner.

Catching up on paperwork

You may get a little behind on this to start off with, since you will be getting used to a new routine. Hopefully, your backlog will not become substantial, and you should be able to keep it to a minimum by developing a suitable procedure for administration.

Reviewing administrative procedure

In a similar way to reviewing case histories, you need to review your administration from time to time. This will enable you to see what has worked and what has not, and make suitable adjustments.

Initially the work involved in administration may not be too onerous, but it is important to keep on top of it. If you take time to organize your time while your business builds, this preparation will not only result in an ability to manage the endless small tasks that are needed to keep your business running efficiently when you become busy, but also make you aware of the opportunities presented by good planning, preparation and education.

Re-examining your business plan

It is a good idea to do this every few weeks as it gives you a sense of how your business is progressing and whether you may be overspending. This constant reappraisal allows you to adjust the way you are handling your money.

Businesses only remain successful by being very aware of the environment around them and adapting to it. You may not be busy enough because you have misjudged your locality, but if you have logically worked through and researched writing a business plan this should not occur.

What you can do when you are able to leave the clinic

General networking

This is where you develop links with people other than patients. These people could be responsible for sending patients to you, so you need to develop a productive working relationship with them. They can vary from your suppliers or local shopkeepers, to other therapists, practice managers, or GPs.

Contact can be maintained in several ways:

- Face-to-face contact.
- Telephone.
- Letters.
- Emails.

It takes some fine-tuning to gauge what type of contact is appropriate, since this will vary from person to person.

Networking between therapists

Networking is crucial for developing a good practice. It cannot help towards achieving the best treatment for your patient but may result in a steady flow of referrals. Colleague referral is obviously much easier in a well-run multidisciplinary practice, but not impossible as a sole practitioner.

That a patient may be seeing two practitioners for the same problem is not unheard of. It is a matter of creating an alliance for the sake of the patient. For example, the teaming of a chiropractor and a remedial masseur works well for a patient, as the chiropractor usually cannot perform the type of deep massage that can be achieved by the masseur. Conversely, the remedial masseur is not qualified to manipulate a patient.

Patients always appreciate honesty and a practitioner who shows a genuine interest in their welfare.

It may also be possible for two practitioners of the same discipline to see the same patient at different times. This form of networking allows for more flexible working hours so that if you are not available at certain times for treatment your colleague may be, and vice versa.

Conclusion

The initial period of running your own business is usually a strange combination of anxiety at plunging into the unknown, exhaustion while trying to perform two jobs, each pulling on your time, and periods of frustration when patients do not seem to be filling the clinic quickly enough.

Strangely, when practitioners look back on this time they see it as one of the most stimulating and exciting times in their lives, since it provided them with the steepest learning curve they had ever experienced.

Useful website

http://www.bnf.org

British National Formulary

Reference

Covey SR, Merrill AR, Merrill RR 1999 First things first. Simon and Schuster, New York

How to deal with money matters now your clinic is open

22

Chapter contents

Once your clinic is under way, managing your finances can be a little tricky until you have adjusted to your new way of life.

Practitioners who are setting up their own clinic for the first time and have never before run their own business usually come from one of two categories:

- Those who have been employees and have received a wage with all the deductions removed.
- Those who have been self-employed but working as practitioners in other clinics.

On many occasions, the new practitioner has been used to a much higher income and has to adjust to a lower level for an initial period, and therefore reduced expenditure. At the same time, money is suddenly going out of the account for more than everyday living expenses, because there are also unaccustomed running costs of a clinic. It is this combination of reduced income and overspending that starts to create a problem.

It can take time to adjust to the amount of money required for the everyday running of your clinic and being unable to have the usual amount of ready cash to spend. Even if there is a surprising surplus, it is important to build up a suitable amount of cash in case you need access to money quickly for an emergency.

Recognizing financial problems and controlling them should not be a problem if you have put together a business plan and have your cash-flow and profit/loss forecast to hand. Although a cash-flow and profit/loss forecast is an estimate, it is none the less a useful guideline to keep you focused on managing your money.

The basics

These are just a continuation of the clinic administration protocol.

Check all paid invoices against your bank statements. Do make sure that all cheques you have signed have the recipient and a brief note of what they were for written legibly on the stub. There is nothing worse for you or your accountant if you cannot remember whom you paid and what for, or finding that even you are unable to read the cheque stub.

Staple cash receipts for small items into your bankbook, or store them somewhere they are easily accessible.

Spreading the cost

Direct debits can be used to pay for such items as membership fees, insurance, and advertisements in *Yellow Pages*. They also prevent you missing an important payment where your membership might be at risk if you do not pay on time. It is important, however, to keep an eye on these, because if they are not correctly cancelled you will find money continues to go out of your account. Recovery of this money is relatively simple, but will not be immediate, which might create problems with your cash flow.

Dealing with the bank

Communication with your bank is very important if you think you may be overrunning your overdraft facility. Explain the circumstances and how you will resolve it, with a timescale of when the problem is likely to be rectified. Follow this up with a letter. Evasion will only create an air of distrust and will be the equivalent for you of trying to ignore the problem. Communicate with the bank before they communicate with you and deal with problems as quickly as possible.

Quotations

Whenever you have work done, get a written quotation. Often things go wrong and the tradesman concerned may try to pass the cost off onto you. In that case you will have your written quotation.

Check that tradesmen are registered, e.g. plumbers, etc., so that if there is a problem you can approach their association to sort it out.

Prices

Your market research should have ensured that you put a realistic price on your service, but you may at some point have to increase your prices in line with your suppliers increasing theirs. If you do increase your prices, then let people know in advance, probably by a few months, so they are prepared for the change.

Keep the price clear on your literature, or at least inform patients when they ring in.

Do not under-price yourself just to get patients in, or you will work yourself into the ground just to make a basic living. Customers are not always concerned with the price, but with the quality of treatment they are going to get. Those patients who ring round to get quotations of prices are probably the ones who will not appreciate the service you are providing.

It is not advisable to drop your price once you have started or this will send out the wrong message.

There are only three ways to increase the profits of a business:

- Reduce costs.
- Raise prices.
- Increase the number of patients or sales made of goods.

When you have just started out, raising prices is not a possibility for a while. Increasing the numbers of patients will only happen over a period of time. Increasing sales of products is a possibility, but bear in mind that dealing with stock can tie up your money and be financially detrimental if you are not moving it, particularly if the stock is perishable and has a sell-by date.

Check the code of ethics of your professional body, as it is possible you may not be allowed to earn more in sales of goods than you are in treatments.

At the end of the day you are usually left with the first option, which is to reduce costs, which may well put your private income under stress for a period of time.

Financial forecasting

At first, the cash-flow and profit/loss forecast is a prediction, but as time goes on you will be able to monitor your performance against it.

Your projections and the reality of your business progress rarely match completely, but measuring actual against budget on a regular basis will enable you to adjust quickly to meet any change in circumstances.

Variances may be due to:

- Reduction in patients.
- Increase in expenditure due to rises in costs of services, insurance, etc.
- Interest rates being higher than expected.
- Overspending, e.g. on expensive holidays, clothes, gadgets, etc.

The forecast also helps you to predict income and expenses over a period of time and see when certain outgoings are going to occur. This is very important, as some expenses will have to be paid up in advance.

Accounts

There is a danger in a business that has a part cash element of making genuine mistakes with the recording of cash. Extra care and greater transparency of accounting is therefore necessary for cash transactions to avoid HM Revenue & Customs getting the wrong impression. In the unfortunate event of you being chosen, at random, for an investigation by HM Revenue & Customs you will need to account for every penny, and they are very thorough.

A ledger (Figs 22.1 and 22.2) is a very useful item to have and can be filled in whenever money is put into the bank or goes out of the clinic in the form of cheques or cash. The system is simple to use and self-explanatory. 'Drawings' is the amount of money you take out of your business for personal use.

You may wish to keep a separate book for small cash items such as purchasing tea or coffee.

While you are starting up, unless you are very confident with using computer accounting packages, use a cashbook system for bookkeeping. Not only are your bookkeeping requirements likely to be very simple, but

	Month				
Gross takings	Other	Bankings	Net takings	Cash payments	Drawings

Figure 22.1 Example of entries for bookkeeping: left-hand side of ledger.

	Month						
Wages	Services	Advertising	Stationery	Equipment	Professional fees	Consumables	Sundries

Figure 22.2 Example of entries for bookkeeping: right-hand side of ledger.

many accountants feel that computer accounting packages in the hands of the uninitiated are more trouble than they are worth. One wrong entry can create a whole series of errors which can take some time to trace back to its cause.

If you have an employee, make sure that your records of PAYE and National Insurance are up to date. If you are not confident in this or any other aspect of bookkeeping, then bring someone in who is. Unless you run an empire of clinics, it is likely that your accounts will be recorded in a simple ledger of incomings and outgoings, which a competent bookkeeper will be able to organize for you.

Credit control

Usually this is not a problem. Health insurance companies are very reliable in paying up although it can take up to 3 weeks or more for you to be paid. Paying directly into you bank account by BACS does speed things up.

It is usually not a good idea to allow accounts unless the patient is long-standing and reliable. Unfortunately, pursuing non-payment through small claims courts is never very fruitful for a self-employed practitioner. Such courts take a part of the settlement for expenses, so at the end of the day you may have lost more money by pursuing this path, as you will have to take the day off work. Occasionally, however, you may have to go through the process on principle. For example, if you work in a small town or a small community where word gets round fast, it may be necessary to use a small claims court to let it be known that people cannot get away with not paying their bills. Fortunately people who exploit this situation are very rare.

Bouncing cheques

Unfortunately, a cheque card is no assurance of payment. If there is no money left in the bank account and the overdraft limit has been exceeded, then it is very possible for the bank not to honour the cheque.

It is usual to incur a bank charge for a cheque that has not been honoured. This should be added to the final bill when the patient pays.

Not turning up for appointments

It is probably a good idea to have some sort of notice, either on the wall of the reception area or on the business card that you give to patients, saying that unkept appointments will have to be paid for. This shows that you mean business, and ensures that a patient who has failed to keep an appointment will be unlikely to do so again.

Conclusion

Finances always cause the most grief to the new practitioner, and if you do not get to grips with this area quickly, then you will have great difficulty in doing so later.

Your bookkeeping should be simple, as most practitioners start on a low budget and without staff.

Providing you are conscientious and methodical you will be able to keep up to date with your financial transactions and ultimately refer to your cash-flow and profit/loss forecasts to see how you are performing. This will ultimately enable you to adjust your budget accordingly and stay financially viable.

What about the future?

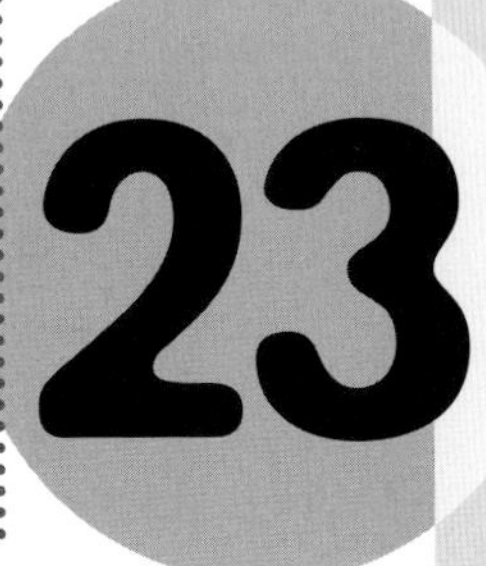

The only right way to run a business is to ensure that at the end of the day you can make a living out of it and that your lifestyle is the right one for you.

The complementary field is ideally suited for expression of individuality. Some practitioners, once they have built up a respectable practice, are happy with a modest income, while others seek expansion. Both types of practice provide exactly the same expertise and job satisfaction in entirely different surroundings, and each works because of the personality of the practitioner. Success, therefore, must be based on the degree of life satisfaction.

Once you have reached a stage where you are up to capacity, you will have to make a decision about whether to stay as you are or grow. For some practitioners this can be as difficult as the first time they established their own clinic, whereas others have always possessed a clear picture of where they are going in life. This is why it is important before you start your first clinic that you have some sort of life map in place, so these types of crossroads do not come as a surprise.

If you choose to expand, then following the principles laid out in this book will guide you. A larger clinic is just the same in concept as opening a new clinic, but on a larger scale with a few more considerations. This time the financial risk is higher, but you will have already been through the process before, so you will not be venturing into the unknown. You will need to plan in exactly the same way as you did on starting your first business. Market research and financial planning with a view to a business plan and keeping to your budget will be just as vital.

Opening up your own clinic will be the biggest step in your business career and as a practitioner. The experience you acquire in doing so is invaluable for making further business decisions and creating growth in you on a more personal level.

Starting your own clinic is a remarkable milestone in your life. No matter how big or small it is, you will be in charge of your own enterprise and solely responsible for the direction you take it in. It is an exciting time, so make the most of it and enjoy it.

Index

C

D

N

O

P

Q

R

S

T

U

V

W

X

Y